Preventing Patient Falls

SECOND EDITION

T0178029

Janice M. Morse, PhD (Nurs), PhD (Anthro), FAAN, is a professor and the Barnes Presidential Endowed Chair at the College of Nursing, University of Utah. She was previously a professor, Faculty of Nursing, and the Founder, Director and Scientific Director of the International Institute for Qualitative Methodology at the University of Alberta, Canada, and professor at The Pennsylvania State University. With doctorates in both nursing and anthropology, Dr. Morse conducts research, funded by NIH and CIHR, into suffering and comforting, as well as developing qualitative research methods. She also serves as a consultant for Hill Rom Industries. She has published extensively in the area of falls, and is author of the *Morse Fall Scale* and serves as editor of *Qualitative Health Research* and was founding co-editor of *International Journal of Qualitative Methods*. She is the co-author of the *Morse Fall Scale,* and has authored, coauthored or edited 14 books including: *Preventing Patient Falls* (1997), and has many publications on identifying fall risk and protecting the fall-prone patient. Dr. Morse has honorary doctorates from the University of Newcastle, Australia and Athabasca University (Canada) for her contributions to nursing science.

Preventing Patient Falls

Establishing a Fall Intervention Program

SECOND EDITION

JANICE M. MORSE, PhD (Nurs), PhD (Anthro), FAAN

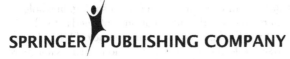

SPRINGER PUBLISHING COMPANY

New York

Springer Publishing Company, LLC
11 West 42nd Street
New York, NY 10036
www.springerpub.com

Acquisitions Editor: Allan Graubard
Project Manager: Barbara A. Chernow
Cover design: Joanne E. Honigman
Composition: Agnew's, Inc.

08 09 10 11 12/ 5 4 3 2 1

Library of Congress Cataloging-in-Publication Data

Morse, Janice M.
   Preventing patient falls : establishing a fall intervention program / Janice M. Morse. — 2nd ed.
      p. ; cm.
   Includes bibliographical references and index.
   ISBN 978-0-8261-0389-5
   1. Health facilities—Safety measures. 2. Falls (Accidents)—Prevention. I.Title.
[DNLM: 1. Accidental Falls—prevention & control. 2. Safety Management. 3. Health Facilities. WX 185 M886p 2009]
   RA969.9.M67   2009
   613′.0438—dc22

                                                                    2008037759

Printed in the United States of America by Malloy.

The author and the publisher of this Work have made every effort to use sources believed to be reliable to provide information that is accurate and compatible with the standards generally accepted at the time of publication. Because medical science is continually advancing, our knowledge base continues to expand. Therefore, as new information becomes available, changes in procedures become necessary. We recommend that the reader always consult current research and specific institutional policies before performing any clinical procedure. The author and publisher shall not be liable for any special, consequential, or exemplary damages resulting, in whole or in part, from the readers' use of, or reliance on, the information contained in this book.

   The publisher has no responsibility for the persistence or accuracy of URLs for external or third-party Internet Web sites referred to in this publication and does not guarantee that any content on such Web sites is, or will remain, accurate or appropriate.

For my Mother
Avis Hazel Blake Lambourne
Who never falls—
but, as a physiotherapist, is
always concerned

Contents

Contents

Preface

In 1982, when I took my first position as a clinical nurse researcher at the University of Alberta Hospitals, I was asked to "look at" the problem of patient falls on the rheumatology unit, a 32-bed unit that was used as a demonstration unit for nursing research. A quick look at the fall rate in that unit showed that if I were to conduct a research project of patient falls in that unit, it would take me 32 years to collect enough data. This is an important fact for everyone planning to implement a fall intervention project—a patient fall is a relatively rare event, and if you consider the fall rate over a short period of time—perhaps 1 month—in a patient care unit, you find that the fall rate is unstable. That is, it goes up and down, and if you have one patient that falls repeatedly—three times in 24 hours, for instance—that patient's fall incidents will really inflate your records. This does not mean that you should not watch your fall rate, only that you should not focus on the fall rate for a unit over a short period of time, letting the fall rate accrue over 12 monthly periods.

I accepted the challenge "to look at falls", and this started a research program that still continues. First, we did as most researchers do: we conducted a chart review of all patient falls for 1 year. This provided us with an institutional profile of falls, a baseline fall rate, and enabled us to show the hospital that falls were indeed a serious problem. Next, we obtained funding to conduct a prospective study of falls—and we examined 100 patients who fell at the time of the fall, and 100 controls. From this study we developed the *Morse Fall Scale (MFS)*, and by examining the errors (the false positives and false negatives), we identified three types of falls—*anticipated physiological falls, unanticipated physiological falls,* and *accidental falls*—reclassifying the previous system of *instrinsic* and *extrinsic falls*, and manipulated the data set on the computer to determine the reliability and validity of the *MFS*. Next, we were interested in the clinical feasibility of the *MFS*, and we conducted a prospective study in three clinical settings: a nursing home, a medical center, and a rehabilitation hospital. We prepared a video so that nurses could have standardized training in the use of the *Scale*, and we provided data collection sheets. Nurses in 6 patient care areas rated all patients daily. At this time, about 1985, there were very few fall intervention strategies. Nurses tried to watch patients carefully, and often patients were allowed to sit close to the nursing stations in the daytime, or nurses would bring patient beds out to these areas at night, or ask relatives to come and sit with the patients. Nurses restrained patients very frequently, with a waist restraint, and sometimes with wrist restraints as well; patients were secured in a gerichair with a locked tray, so they could not slide or get out; patients usually had a vest or waist restraint while in a wheelchair. Nurses caring for restless patients made an innovative bed alarm, by pinning the call bell to the patients nightshirt—a risky practice—so that when the patient climbed out of bed, the call bell would pull out of the wall and the emergency call bell systems would be activated.

The problem at the time was that the *MFS* was good at predicting who was likely to fall, but did not indicate what to do to protect the patient. I was very afraid that if we introduced the *Scale*—naively believing that it would be immediately adopted—that restraint use would dramatically increase.

Therefore, at that time, my research program shifted to fall interventions and how to determine if we could care for patients without restraints. A bioengineering team and I developed a bed alarm and obtained a patent for one made out of a blood pressure cuff. We placed the alarm on a bed with three-quarter length side rails, to let the patient have a safe route out of the bed, and inflated the cuff. When the patient moved out of the bed across the inflated cuff, an air pressure switch sounded an alarm. This primitive alarm was so successful that the nurses would not let us take the alarm away, so we improved it: prototype II had 2 metal plates and a spring, so that it would self inflate between uses.

With the bioengineers, I also developed the specs for a low bed, believing that injuries could be reduced if patients had less distance to fall; we also received a patent for that work. Meanwhile, we tested more comfortable wheelchairs, and the Ambularm©—a battery alarm with a mercury switch which was placed on the patient's thigh, so that when the patient stood, the alarm sounded.

But the most important project I did in this period was to determine if patients could be cared for without restraints. I chose to do this work in a 24-bed psycho-geriatric unit, in which 22 of the 24 patients were restrained. I took the proposal over to the unit and began applications for funding. Unfortunately, the proposal was not funded on the first application. Much of my time was spent persuading the medical committee that collecting the data using videotape and using ethology as the method was not only the safest way to do this research, but the only way to answer the research questions. When I finally had received the funding, I went over to the unit to tell the nurses that the project would start, they said, "You know Jan, that was such a great idea that we have taken all of the restraints off!" I do believe this is an illustration of the fact that you do not have to do research to implement change—just to threaten to do it. Actually, the unit still had four patients in restraints, those considered incorrigible, and it was from these four that we selected two patients for our project. The project was a success, and it was conducted at the same time that the *Releasing Restraints* movement started, led by a Quaker group in Philadelphia.

These studies were published, the MFS studies published, and at the same time, a number of bed alarms and other fall intervention devices, such as bed mats, became available. I considered my work finished and moved on to other things.

But the fall research did not go away. Nurses trying to implement a fall intervention program kept calling with questions. My greatest concern was that the depth of research pertaining to falls was not being examined, and only the publications pertaining to the *MFS* were being used. By 1997, I had published *Preventing Patient Falls* (Sage), and the fall conferences (sponsored by the VISN 8 Safety Center) began, providing an important annual forum for the discussion of fall research.

Still, the questions kept coming, and it became clear that the *MFS* was often misapplied. Although I thought I had been clear that to use the *MFS*, one had to observe the patient at the time of scoring, to record gait, and to ask the patient questions in order to measure mental status, I kept learning of studies in which the *MFS* was evaluated by using chart data. I still do not know how it is possible to get a score from chart data! Also, nurses used the *Scale* as a category of 3 classes—high risk, medium risk and low risk, rather than using the score itself. Furthermore, even though I had produced a reliable and valid scale, research nurses in hospitals everywhere started producing their own "home made" scales (with no reliability or validity) and often with scores that were estimated using their best judgment, rather than scores derived from the research itself. This was such a puzzle to me. It was also disconcerting that the studies evaluating the *MFS* by scoring all patients in the unit and then recording who fell and who did not fall, forgot that if a patient was recorded as at risk of falling, fall intervention strategies to prevent the fall should be immediately implemented. What these studies are measuring is not the efficacy of the *MFS*, but the efficacy of the fall interventions!

How did nursing research get into such a mess? I have several ideas—nursing education had been fast and furiously teaching nurses to be researchers at the baccalaureate and masters level—teaching them some principles of research, enough for them to want to do research, but with not enough knowledge to do it well. In this situation, such research could place both the patient and the hospital in jeopardy!

So, this book is my second attempt to clear up all the grey areas in patient fall intervention programs. I hope I have done a better job this time. Please keep asking questions, for it helps me understand where I have not been clear, or where I have left a gap in my explanations.

Janice Morse
2008

Acknowledgments

I have many people to thank—people who have been an integral part of the research team, who have assisted or encouraged me. First, I thank my collaborators: Nora Morrow, Gail Federspeil, Margaret Prowse, Susanne Tylko, Robert Morse, Herb Dixon, Colleen Black, Kathy Oberle, Julian Stedman, Pat Donahue, Edna McHutchion, Mary Watson, Charlotte Pooler, and Pierre Gervais. This research was funded by the University of Alberta Hospitals Foundation, the Glenrose Hospital, Edmonton, Alberta, and the "bed" project by Hill Rom Industries. I thank Hill Rom Industries, Rick Barker and Penny Gilbert for their support of the fall program, their development of the training DVD and the web site, and their support of my many visits to hospitals to consult on patient falls.

I am grateful for the permission to reprint previously published material from:

Canadian Journal of Public Health
The Gerontologist
Canadian Journal on Aging
Social Science & Medicine
QRB: Quality Review Bulletin
The Annual Review of Nursing Research
Research in Nursing and Health
Canadian Journal for Nursing Research

This book is dedicated to my mother, a physiotherapist of the old school, who believes in massage, heat, and exercise and that patient falls are preventable!

Preventing Patient Falls

1

Creating a Fall Intervention Program: An Overview

Once considered an "accident," an unavoidable problem of illness, disability, or the frailty of advancing age, patient falls were accepted as a normal consequence of illness or aging, and any injury resulting from the fall was accepted simply as "bad luck." Over the past three decades, research has developed to the point where we are able to predict which patients are likely to fall from the frailty of illness and aging (called an *anticipated physiological fall*) and to implement strategies to prevent the fall (i.e., *preventative strategies*) or to protect the patient from injury (i.e., *protective strategies*) should a serious fall occur. As the majority of falls that occur within the hospital may be classified as *anticipated physiological falls*, this research is making an important contribution to the prevention of iatrogenic injuries or even death.

Does this mean that falls are never accidental? No—a person who has none of the characteristics that indicate fall-proneness may have a true accident—for instance, they may slip on spilled water or something greasy on the floor or trip on a step or on even their own footwear. But those who are rated as fall-prone **do not** have accidents, because we *expect* them to trip or slip. Because these patients have a poor gait, impaired balance, are cognitive impaired, and do not use their walking aids correctly, we expect them to trip or to slip, to lose their balance, and to fall. In other words, they are an "accident about to happen," and it is the responsibility of caregivers to ensure the safety of those who score as fall-prone on the fall screening tools.

On the other hand, accidental falls only "happen" to those who do not score at risk of falling. For this reason, the second type of fall, *accidental falls*, are relatively uncommon, typically comprising only of 14% of all falls in hospital.

The third type of fall that occurs in hospitals is the *unanticipated physiological fall*. This occurs when a person with none of the risk factors falls because of a seizure, because they suddenly feel faint, or because a knee "suddenly gave way." The first fall of this type cannot be predicted, but our role is to provide protection from injury should the fall reoccur.

Falls in hospitals occur at amazingly similar rates among institutions. But this does not mean that an institution cannot improve its fall rate. This book presents two decades of research into patient falls in a form that is useful to hospital administrators, physicians, and nurses.

> Standardized fall rates assist clinicians in evaluating a fall prevention program by comparing fall rates with other institutions.

The main purpose is to consolidate a research program into patient falls and make the research clinically applicable by presenting it in a form that is useful to hospital administrators and nurses. However, the primary objective is to provide instruction on how to develop a program using the *Morse Fall Scale* (*MFS*).

In Chapter 2, I discuss how to make your environment as safe as possible to minimize accidental falls. This should always be the first task undertaken before one begins a formal fall intervention program. Then, in Chapter 3 I discuss how to prepare your institution administratively for a fall intervention program. I will discuss how to collect baseline data, so that falls are monitored on an ongoing basis, and you will be able to evaluate the reduction of falls once your program is in place. I will show you how to use fall data proactively to identify "hot spots"—areas in which falls occur repeatedly—and to then rectify problems to reduce your fall rate even further.

Some patients fall repeatedly—*multiple fallers* or *repeat fallers*—and frequently the second fall occurs at the same time of day while the patient is doing the same activity. Prevention includes a "warning" system to alert the staff to his fall pattern, so that the second and subsequent fall can be intercepted.

Chapter 4 reviews how to identify the fall prone patient—those who are at risk of an *anticipated physiological fall* and how to score a patient for fall risk using the *MFS*. Chapter 5 focuses on fall *prevention* strategies—interventions that will prevent a fall from occurring—and fall *protective* strategies—intervention that will minimize patient injury should a fall occur. Fall *assessment* will be then discussed in Chapter 7; Chapter 8 reviews how to assess the effectiveness of your program.

These components, taken together, make your fall program solid. Initially, each step must be implemented sequentially, but once the program begins, you must attend to each area and keep each component intact. Throughout the book, I will address questions that have been asked about fall intervention programs and the use of the *Scale*.

The second section contains Appendices that present all of the research information on the *Scale*—how the instrument was developed, how to determine the level of risk, and what norms to expect, as well as foreign translations of the *Scale*.

Despite recent advances in our understanding of patient falls, they remain a major problem. Falls have been identified as the second leading cause of accidental death in the United States, and 75% of those falls occur in the elderly population. When hospitalized, patients are placed in double jeopardy. In addition to the hazards of everyday living and of aging, they are weakened from illness, surgery, and bed rest; they may feel unwell and unsteady as a result of receiving multiple medications; they may experience conditions that force them to rush to the bathroom, such as urinary frequency or urgency or diarrhea; they are placed in a strange environment where the furniture is arranged differently and is dis-

> Six percent of patient falls result in serious injuries that further compromise health status or even result in death.

concertingly disproportionate; and, they must rely on asking strangers for assistance with intimate and embarrassing bodily functions.

However, it is not the fall rate of hospitalized patients that is important, but the injury rate. Six percent of patient falls in the hospital result in serious injuries that further compromise health status or even result in death, either from the fall or from secondary causes. Injuries from falls dramatically increase health care costs by an estimated billions of dollars annually (Jasson, Stenback, Leifman et al., 2004). Of greater concern, falls in the hospital may result in death from a fractured skull, or 6 weeks after a fall that results in a fractured hip as a result of a secondary cause, such as pneumonia.

THE PROBLEM OF PATIENT FALLS

What is a fall? One of the problems in conducting fall research is defining exactly what a fall is, so that clinicians know when and what to report as a fall, resulting in some consistency in fall rates and in fall research. Morris and Isaacs (1980) define a fall as "an untoward event in which the patient comes to rest unintentionally on the floor." But this definition remains problematic for clinicians. Has the patient fallen *if* the patient is "caught" and lowered into a chair? Is it considered a fall if the patient grabs a handrail and does not land on the floor? And is it considered a fall if a nurse finds a patient on the floor, but the patient cannot tell the nurse what happened, and the event was not witnessed? My only advice is to use your best judgment. It seems to me that all the scenarios described above may be considered a fall, but not necessarily reported as such. Report the witnessed fall that was not witnessed, but the patient whose fall was intercepted by the nurse or the one who grabbed the handrail were "near misses." Near misses must be recorded—for next time there may be a real fall— but are not reported as incidents and do not enter the fall database. The golden rule for determining what is a fall is based upon the fall screening tools which measure the likelihood of falling from a standing position while walking or getting out of bed to stand. If other miscellaneous incidents are entered into the fall database, then the lowering of your institution's fall rate may be very frustrating.

However, the problem of what is and is not a reportable fall is compounded with the inclusion of toddlers, who fall in the normal developmental stages of learning to walk, or who may climb and fall from a height on to the floor. Neither of these instances is considered a reportable fall—so it makes no sense to score toddler or young children with a fall scale. The fall risk scales measure adult risk of falling while walking, and care must be taken to prevent these incidents. But those interventions to prevent toddlers from falling are different from the interventions that are developed for the adult fall scales. Using, for instance, the *MFS* with toddlers and young children is a waste of time. The *Scale* was not developed for such use, and the scores will be meaningless.

One last source of errors in the fall data includes patients who are dropped. A nurse told me that they were turning an unconscious patient, they forgot to put the side rail up and the patient "fell" on to the floor. This patient has not fallen, but has been dropped. This incident should not be in the fall database—hospitals must develop an "other" database for such instances. Dropped occurrences may also occur in pediatrics. Nurses have reported that sometimes a mother may fall asleep while holding her infant, and the infant may "fall" or slide on to the floor. Again, this infant has been dropped, and this incident should not be recorded as a fall. It is a reportable incident, but it is not a fall.

It is incredibly important to **report all falls.** The reason is that once the patient has fallen, s/he is particularly likely to fall a second time. Furthermore, the odds are that the patient will fall a second time doing the same thing. Thus, while the most important aspect of prevention is to predict the fall before it occurs, it is also important to examine and record the circumstances surrounding each fall, so that reoccurrence may be prevented.

> Examine and record the circumstances surrounding the fall, so that a reoccurrence may be prevented.

Falls occur in all types of health care institutions, to all patient populations *except* patients who are unconscious and infants who cannot stand. Table 1.1 shows fall rates for some types of patient populations. Notice that the rates vary according to the patient care setting. They

Table 1.1

COMPARISON OF PATIENT FALL RATES[1] AND INJURY RATES FOR VARIOUS PATIENT POPULATIONS

AUTHOR (DATE)	SETTING	FALL RATE (# FALLS/# PATIENT BED DAYS) × 1,000	INJURY RATE	COMMENTS
Barnett (2002)	General hospital	9.6	22%	England
Healey et al. (2004)	Geriatric	17.99	4.42/ 1000 pt bed days	England
Hitcho et al. (2004)	Medical Neurology	6.12 6.12	8%	USA
Schwendiman (2008)	Geriatrics Internal medicine Surgery	10.7 9.6 3.2	30.1% minor 5.1% major	Switzerland
von Rentein-Kruse et al. (2007)	General	10.0	26.9%	Germany

[1]Unless otherwise stated, patient fall rate = (# falls/# patient bed days) × 1,000

are lowest in the general, acute care hospitals and highest in the nursing homes, with the rates in the rehabilitation hospital falling somewhere in between. Within the hospital, there is variation among units, with the lowest rate in obstetrics and higher fall rates in gerontology, psychiatry, and rehabilitation units. These rates are important because they give the clinician some basis for comparison as the rates in one's own institution are recorded and better understood. In reality, however, a fall is a fairly uncommon event. This means that the statistics can be easily inflated if a fall rate is estimated for a small group (such as a unit) for a short period of time. As I mentioned previously, several falls (or one patient falling repeatedly) could inflate the fall rate, and we see this phenomena in some of the statistics below (see Kilpack et al., 1991). When the patient population is increased (as with reporting on the entire hospital, especially over the period of a year or more), then the fall rate becomes more stable. Another important point is that when a program is first initiated, the fall rates *escalate* because of enthusiastic reporting by staff members.

For this reason it is also important to record *injury rates*. While an injury is a much rarer event, a fall that results in an injury is always reported. Thus injury rates tend to be more reliable and, therefore, more stable than fall rates. This aspect of recording will be discussed later.

> When a fall prevention program is first initiated, fall rates *escalate* because of increased reporting.

IDENTIFYING TYPES OF FALLS

Patients fall for a variety of reasons, and if falls are to be prevented, it is critical to understand the etiology of a fall.[1] Analysis of circumstances surrounding 100 patients who fell and 100 randomly selected patients who had not fallen (Morse, Tylko, & Dixon, 1987) revealed that three types of patient falls occurred in hospitals and long-term care institutions.

Because falls have different causes, the strategies for preventing patient falls are different for each type of fall. A fall may be classified as *accidental* or *physiological,* with the physiological falls further classified as predictable—that is, an *anticipated physiological fall* (i.e. the patient exhibits signs that indicates the likelihood of falling and scores at risk on the *MFS*) or as unpredictable—that is, an *unanticipated physiological fall.*

> Identifying falls as *anticipated physiological falls, unanticipated physiological falls,* or *accidental falls* is important, because methods for prediction and prevention differ for each type of fall.

---

[1] Authors previously sorted falls into two categories: *intrinsic* and *extrinsic* causes (Morris and Isaacs, 1980). *Intrinsic* factors are those caused by the patient's illness or condition, such as a stroke or an amputation. *Extrinsic* factors are those caused by the environment, such as factors causing the patient to slip or to trip.

Accidental Falls

Fourteen percent of all falls are considered accidental, caused by the patient slipping, tripping, or having some other mishap. These falls are often caused by environmental factors, such as spilled water or urine on the floor. A patient may fall when using an IV stand for support if the wheels stick suddenly, or they may fall when the top of the IV pole catches on an overhead curtain railing or doorway. Alternatively, the patient may fall when climbing out of bed, if the bed is in an unexpectedly high position. Accidental falls may also be caused by the patient making errors of judgment, such as leaning against a curtain, thinking it was a supportive wall; misjudging the width of a doorway and not realizing that the doorways in institutions are wider than those in the home; or leaning on a bedside locker when the locker suddenly rolls away. Accidental falls may also occur if the patient loses balance when ambulating. For instance, the patient may be rising from a chair and reaching for a walker, leaning from the bed and reaching for an object, using poor technique when transferring, or forgetting to lift the foot pedal of the wheelchair before standing. It is important to note that the patient who experiences an accidental fall may not have been identified as being at risk of falling on the MFS.

> Fourteen percent of all falls are considered *accidental*, caused by the patient slipping, tripping, or having some other mishap.

> Anticipated physiological falls (78% of falls) occur when residents who score "at risk of falling" on the *MFS* subsequently fall.

Because accidental falls are not due to physical factors but are rather caused by environmental hazards or errors of judgment, prevention strategies are designed to ensure that the environment is free from hazards, that the patient is oriented to the environment, and has received instruction on how to use walkers, and so forth. This includes instruction on the correct method of transferring from a wheelchair.

Anticipated Physiological Falls

These are falls that occur with the patients identified as fall-prone by scoring "at risk of falling" on the *MFS*. The items on the *MFS* are based on research findings and represent six factors that contribute significantly to the patient's likelihood of falling (Morse, Morse, & Tylko, 1989). These factors include more than one diagnosis (and thus is in the index for polypharmacy), a previous fall, a weak or impaired gait, the lack of a realistic assessment of his or her own abilities to go to the bathroom unassisted, an IV or saline lock, and an ambulatory aid. Anticipated physiological falls constitute 78% of all falls.

UNANTICIPATED PHYSIOLOGICAL FALLS

These are falls that may be attributed to physiological causes, but are created by conditions that **cannot be predicted** before the first occurrence. They constitute approximately 8% of all falls. Examples of physiological conditions that result in unanticipated physiological falls include seizures, "drop attacks," fainting, or a pathological fracture of the hip. Depending on the cause, when this type of fall occurs—and there is a likelihood that the underlying condition may recur—nursing attention is targeted toward either preventing a second fall or preventing injury when the patient falls again. For example, nurses may teach a patient with orthostatic hypotension how to recognize the dizziness on rising, and how to get up slowly, thereby reducing the risk of falling.

> *Unanticipated physiological falls* may be attributed to physiological causes that **cannot be predicted** before the first fall.

Summary

Differentiating falls into anticipated and unanticipated physiological falls and accidental falls is important because methods for prediction and prevention differ for each type of fall. The *MFS* predicts *physiological anticipated falls*. Prevention strategies include developing an individualized fall prevention program that will lower the patient's risk score and prevent the fall. *Accidental falls* cannot be predicted using the *Scale*. They are prevented by making the environment as safe as possible.

Unanticipated physiological falls cannot be predicted using the *Scale* nor can they be prevented from occurring the first time. Prevention is targeted toward strategies for protecting the patient from a second fall. The notion of *protection* is important, because sometimes the fall cannot be prevented. Rather, protection strategies are taken to ensure the patient does not injury him/herself in the fall. For example, a patient with epilepsy may fall in the process of having a seizure, and this cannot be predicted or changed. But the protective strategy would be to teach that patient how to protect his head or to ensure that the patient wears a helmet to prevent head injury should a seizure occur. Many patients such as those with Parkinson's disease, can be taught *how* to fall.

> The *MFS* predicts physiological anticipated falls.

COLLECTING BASELINE DATA

The first step, before making the decision to initiate a fall prevention program, is to ascertain how serious the problem of patient falls is in your institution. If falling is a problem, estimate how serious is the problem of *injuries from falls*. The fastest way to evaluate these problems is to analyze the institution's incident report forms used for reporting a fall. Tabulate all falls and injuries that have resulted from a fall over a 12-month period. Calculate the fall rate and the injury rate for your institution using the formula for *fall rate* and *injury rate* presented in Appendix C. If incident report forms are not available for analysis, then it will be necessary to collect fall statistics for a predetermined length of time, preferably for at least 3 months.

Warning: When reviewing the literature containing fall statistics and causes of falls, it is tempting to ignore or "improve" the available screening tools by creating your own fall scale. Sometimes, one chooses items from several scales or one can even select your own items to include in a scale. Such efforts, however, will probably have no reliability or validity and will not be predictive of falling. Save your time and energy by selecting a scale that was developed statistically, preferably using prospective data and NOT chart data. Choose one with reported reliability and validity—one that meets the needs of your institution. You also need to consider its intended use. Altering scale items or altering scale scores will interfere with the scale's reliability and validity. Scales are not created arbitrarily and *must not* be altered.

PLANNING A FALL INTERVENTION PROGRAM

As there are three types of patient falls (an accidental fall, a physiological anticipated fall, and an unanticipated physiological fall), approaches and methods of fall prevention differ with each type of fall. The comprehensive fall prevention program is, therefore, sorted into three components, each targeted to prevent a fall or to protect the patient who is likely to fall.

> The comprehensive fall prevention program is, therefore, sorted into three components, each targeted to prevent a fall or to protect the patient who is likely to fall.

Preventing Accidental Falls

The first type of fall, the accidental fall, is prevented by ensuring a safe environment. This means that the causes of an accidental fall are removed; the process and procedures for checking the environment are described in Chapter 2. While accidental falls may occur in patients with a normal gait, they are more likely to occur in patients who have an abnormal gait. For instance, patients with an impaired gait who

> The accidental fall is prevented by ensuring a safe environment.

shuffle and cannot lift their feet are more likely to trip. Before commencing a fall intervention program, the environmental hazards must be corrected. This includes doing a walk-through with engineering and housekeeping staffs and correcting problems. A safety check must be conducted on all wheelchairs, beds (including brakes and side rails), and walking aides. If it is considered necessary, additional handrails must be installed on the walls. Anything that obstructs the patients' use of these rails (such as trays for charting, glove boxes and hand sanitizers) must be relocated.

Preventing Anticipated Physiological Falls

Anticipated physiological falls are prevented by first identifying who is likely to fall by administering the *MFS*.

Those patients who score at high or medium risk of falling are then assessed to see if the possible cause of the fall may be corrected or lowered. Examples may include altering medications to reduce confusion, using physiotherapy to increase muscle strength and improve gait, or providing correct instructions for the use of a walker, and so forth. Another approach may be to identify a nursing care plan to reduce fall risk, such as waking the patient at night for toileting or increasing surveillance. Alternatively, use bed alarms to assist with patient monitoring should the patient get out of bed without using the call light.

> Anticipated physiological falls are prevented by first identifying who is likely to fall using the *MFS*.

Preventing Unanticipated Physiological Falls

The first *unanticipated physiological fall* cannot be predicted and, therefore, cannot be prevented, because the staff and the patient may not realize that the patient has the condition that precipitates the unexpected fall. That is, the staff may not realize that the patient is seizure-prone until the first seizure occurs. Thus, the intervention is to *protect the patient* by *preventing injury* should a second fall occur. For exam-

> The first *unanticipated patient fall* cannot be prevented— *protect the patient* by preventing injury should a second fall occur.

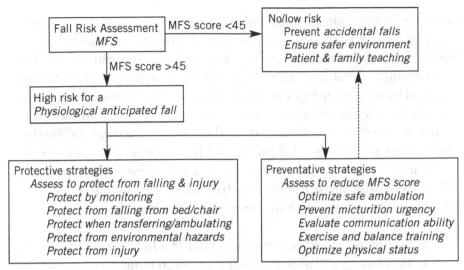

Figure 1.1 Process of Fall Intervention

ple, the patient can be required to wear a helmet to protect against a head injury or hip pads to prevent a fractured hip. A patient with orthostatic hypotension can be taught how to rise from a chair slowly. Each of these approaches is highlighted in Figure 1.1 with references made to the sections that detail each approach.

INSTITUTIONAL COORDINATION FOR FALL PREVENTION

Preventing patient falls requires a planned and coordinated effort. In an institution, this means involving all staff, from the highest level of administration to housekeeping. It includes all health professions, but especially nursing, medicine, pharmacy, and physiotherapy. It includes the records department, risk management, and quality assurance. It includes maintenance workers, such as carpenters and electricians, and it includes administrative staff, such as the Vice President for nursing and area supervisors. Unfortunately, it may even involve the legal department.

The concern of patients who fall is not confined to nursing, and nurses at the bedside must not and cannot solely bear the brunt of responsibility—and the guilt—when patients fall. However, preventing patient falls is a concern that may be spearheaded and coordinated by nursing, and it is an area where leadership in prevention may fall on nursing's shoulders. Most hospitals have a fall program spearheaded by a fall committee, consisting of the head nurses of the units in which falls mainly occur, a quality assurance representative, and sometimes a representative from medicine and pharmacy. While this committee may oversee fall policy and procedures, it is ill equipped to manage the day-to-day nuances of a fall intervention program. *Every hospital must appoint a clinical nurse specialist* to oversee the implementation of the programs. This includes:

- Setting up reporting structures should a fall occur
- Purchasing and allocating fall protection equipment
- Educating staff (and providing ongoing training of newly hired staff) regarding the use of the *MFS* and ongoing monitoring of the program
- Assessing patients who score as high risk or who have fallen for identification of appropriate fall interventions
- Conducting fall assessment and multidisciplinary intervention meetings
- Communicating with housekeeping and engineering
- Communicating with purchasing for fall intervention equipment
- Acting as an intermediary between the fall committee and the staff
- Ongoing monitoring of the fall program, including preparing reports and providing feedback to the committee and staff

There are six basic sequential steps in the establishment of a fall prevention program, and the program should not be implemented until all steps are in place. If one of the steps fails to materialize, then the program should not proceed to implementation. The six steps are illustrated as a flowchart in Figure 1.2.

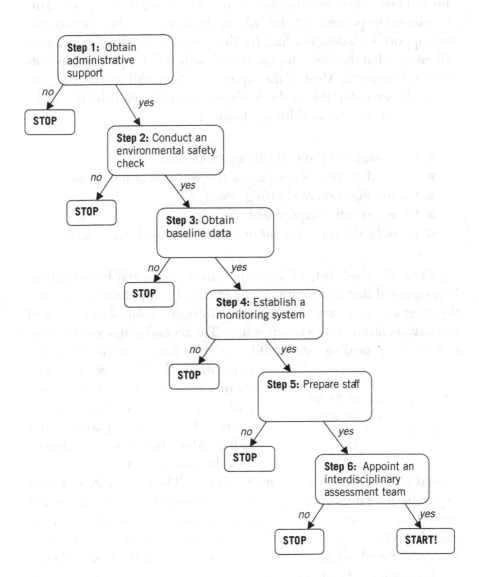

Figure 1.2 Basic administrative steps essential for the successful establishment of a fall intervention program.

Step 1: Obtain Administrative Support

The first task is to develop a plan for implementing the program. This plan should be presented to the administration to obtain commitment and support, including funding, for the program. Briefly, the program will ensure that the environment is optimally safe for patients, as outlined in Chapter 2. Most of the equipment that staff will be suggesting, such as comfortable and safe chairs, should already be available. Funding may be required for the following:

- the position of the Fall Clinical Specialist
- the modification of flooring or the addition of handrails
- the modification of charting systems
- fall intervention equipment
- possibly, the replacement of unsafe beds and mattresses.

From the above list, it is clear that the real cost may be in staffing. It is essential that a clinical nurse specialist be appointed to oversee the program (in a parallel role to the "infection control nurse"), and this may mean creating a new position. The second major and ongoing cost will be providing extra staff to assist on floors once the program is established. When regular staff members are too busy to monitor a patient closely, extra staff may be needed to protect a patient from falling. Many hospitals use "sitters," and the annual cost for sitters may exceed $1,000,000 in a large medical center. The immediate costs are in purchasing safety equipment, such as handrails, bed alarms, or hip protectors. However, these requests are neither exorbitant nor extraordinary: If hospitals are to be accountable for patients' care, then having a safe wheelchair, a bed alarm, and a comfortable seat should not be considered extraordinary.

> Nurses cannot reduce fall rates without funding and support.

It is a serious mistake to implement the use of the fall risk assessment without budgeting for the costs associated with fall intervention. In fact, doing so may place your institution at increased risk for patient falls than not implementing an interventions care plan. Therefore, if Nursing Administration or the Vice President for nursing does not support the program, **DO NOT CONTINUE.** In addition, beginning a program without providing safe interventions places nurses in a helpless position. They will then know that a patient most probably will fall, yet do not have the supports needed to prevent the fall. The only alternative—which is unacceptable—is to restrain the patient—a procedure that will cause harm, further deterioration of the patient's condition, and may be dangerous.

Step 2: Conduct an Environmental Safety Check

Once administration has agreed to support the program, the next step is to conduct a check of each unit to ensure that the environment is safe. This action is also listed previously for the prevention of *accidental falls*. As patients will find it easier to ambulate—and ambulate with more confidence, then they will become stronger (and less likely to experience a physiological fall). Because patients will be able to more safely ambulate without nursing assistance, there will be some savings in staff time.

The newly appointed clinical nurse specialist should, at this time, systematically work through each unit, reviewing with staff which equipment should go for repair, where railings should be installed, and what other furniture or equipment should be purchased or replaced. But until these modifications and repairs have been completed, the program must not commence.

Step 3: Obtain Baseline Data

The third step is to collect statistics on the number of patient falls, specifying the number of falls with injuries, in the institution before the fall prevention program begins. This step may be conducted concurrently with the second step of conducting an environmental safety check. These preintervention statistics are important, for they tell you (1) how serious the problem of patients falls is (and therefore can help you justify the cost of a prevention program); and (2) let you know how effective the program has been for *reducing* falls. That is, to assess the efficacy of the program, "pretest" data must be available for comparison. Available statistics must be checked and compiled in a form that allows for ready comparison.

Step 4: Establish a Monitoring System

Often when a fall prevention program begins, the sudden focus on falls changes nurses' reporting habits. They no longer perceive it as a "punishment" to have to report a fall. Suddenly, "Why did *I* let this patient fall?" becomes, "Why didn't this intervention work?" The removal of blame from the nurse and the change in attitude results in a change of reporting norms. Nurses suddenly report **all** falls, so that the fall rate unexpectedly and, dramatically, increases. Thus, a useful check is to also prepare comparison statistics on the *injury rate* for all injuries that will have been reported. Although *injuries* form a less likely occurrence—and therefore longer periods have to be compared (such as year by year)—they form a more reliable indicator of the value of the program. In addition, it is *prevention of injury* that is the ultimate goal of the program.

> Preventing patient injury is the ultimate goal of the program.

A system for recording the patient's fall score in the patient's chart needs to be developed. In addition, because the patient who falls is extremely likely to fall again during the same period and under the same circumstances, a system for recording the details of each fall must be developed. This record should be kept in a visible place on the unit or should "pop up" on the patient's computer chart. A system of recording and compiling hospital-wide statistics must be developed, so that there is an ongoing check of the fall-prone patients and the high-risk fall areas.

Finally, in conjunction with quality assurance, nursing administration, and the fall committee, decisions need to be made about how and when to score each patient, and how these scores will be recorded. Most importantly, each area needs to determine what score will result in the patient being labeled "at risk of falling" and when fall prevention strategies will be implemented. It is important to note that with the *MFS*, the score may be 25 for moderate risk and 45 for high risk. The methods for making these decisions are presented in Chapter 4. However, it is important that the patient's actual score be listed on the patient's chart and that this score be used when discussing the patient's fall risk.

Step 5: Prepare Staff

By this time, the word should have reached the unit level about the program, and staff training sessions may begin. Staff in-services should be conducted in small groups and consist of:

1 Identify the fall prone patient. Staff training for using the *MFS* is available online from Hill-Rom: *http://www.hill-rom.com/ usa/Safety_PatientFalls.htm.* A CD-Rom is also available—it has better graphics, a more interactive format, and a facilitator's guide for learning verification and certification. The cost is $25USD, order number vt 171ra. Pocket cards of the scale for staff reference are available from Hill-Rom, order number CTG581. Alternatively, small, plastic-covered pocket cards of the *MFS* may be prepared and distributed to staff.

2 Develop a means for identifying fall prevention strategies (see Chapter 5) and the appropriate use of the bed alarms (see Chapter 2).

3 Develop a system for recording the patient's fall score.

4 Develop a system for reporting falls.

5 Develop a protocol for consulting with the "Fall-Nurse" and the fall consultation team.

When holding in-service sessions for staff, present the main methods of preventing falls, the institutional protocol for recording and reporting patient falls, and the protocols for consulting with the fall clinical nurse specialist. A smart idea is to give the unit 2 weeks of "practice" using the *MFS* and recording the scores. In our experience, this allows the staff to become familiar with the *MFS* and become experts at fall assessment before the program formally begins.

Step 6: Appoint an Interdisciplinary Assessment Team

The final step before commencing the program is the appointment of an interdisciplinary team. The role of the team is to combine expertise and consult about "problem" patients who fall repeatedly or are at exceptionally high risk of falling. The team should also periodically review all fall reports and focus especially on institutional patterns. For example, the team may observe that many falls occur in a particular place, and should be able to identify a handrail or some other structural modification that will increase the safety of the area. The team should be chaired by the fall prevention clinical nurse specialist and be composed of a geriatrician, a physical therapist, a pharmacist, and an occupational therapist. Ad hoc members may be added for review of a particular "problem" patient who falls repeatedly. These members may include the patient (if oriented and well enough to attend) or the patient's next of kin, the patient's physician, and the patient's primary nurse.

At the unit level, high-risk cases may be reviewed by nursing staff, with the fall clinical nurse specialist serving as a consultant. Note that the goal of the consultation is to develop a plan to reduce the patient's fall risk score and to develop strategies to prevent a fall. If a fall has occurred, however, focus should be to develop unique and individualized strategies to prevent a reoccurrence.

Only once all of these things are in place, the program can begin.

REFERENCES

Barnett, K. (2002). Reducing patient falls in an acute general hospital. *The Foundations of Nursing Studies, 1*(1), 1–4.

Coussement, J., De Paepe, L., Schwendimann, R., Denhaerynck, K., Dejaeger, E., & Milisen K. (2008). Interventions for preventing falls in acute- and chronic-care hospitals: A systematic review and meta-analysis. *Journal of the American Geriatrics Society, 56*(1), 29–36.

Healey, F., Monro, A., Cockram, A., Adams, V., & Heseltine, D. (2004). Using targeted risk factor reduction to prevent falls in older in-patient: A randomized controlled trial. *Age and Ageing, 33,* 390–395.

Hitcho, E., Krauss, M., Birge, S., Dunagan, W., Fischer, I., Johnson, S., et al. (2004). Characteristics and circumstances of falls in a hospital setting: A prospective analysis. *Journal of General Internal Medicine, 19*(7), 732–739.

Jansson, B., Stenback, M., Leifman, A., & Romelsjo, A. (2004). A small fraction of patients with repetitive injuries account for a large portion of medical costs. *European Journal of Public Health, 14,* 161–167.

Kilpack, V., Boehm, J., Smith, N., & Mudge, B. (1991). Using research-based interventions to decrease patient falls. *Applied Nursing Research, 4*(2), 50–56.

Morris, E. V., & Isaacs, B. (1980). The prevention of falls in geriatric hospital. *Age and Ageing, 9,* 1981–1985.

Morse, J. M., Morse, R. M., & Tylko, S. J. (1989). Development of a scale to identify the fall-prone patient. *Canadian Journal on Aging, 8*(4), 366–377.

Morse, J. M., Tylko, S. J., & Dixon, H. A. (1987). Characteristics of the fall-prone patient. *The Gerontologist, 27*(4), 516–522.

Schwedimann, R., Buhler, H., De Geest, S., & Milisen, K. (2008). Characteristics of hospital inpatient falls across clinical departments. *Gerontology.* DOI: 10.1159/000129954. Published online first. Retrieved June 8, 2008, from http://content.karger.com/produkteDB/produkte.asp?doi=129954

von Renteln-Kruse, W., & Kraus, T. (2007). Incidence of inhospital falls in geriatric patients before and after introduction of an interdisciplinary team-based fall prevention program. *Journal of the American Geriatrics Society, 55,* 2068–2074.

2

Creating a Safe Environment: Preventing Accidental Falls

Ensuring an optimally safe environment will minimize the number of accidental falls in an institution. A safe environment will also reduce the number of potential law suits against the institution, thus indirectly saving staff time and preserving staff morale. It will also build staff morale, because the staff will recognize that the administration supports its goals for a fall-prevention program. This chapter discusses how to create the optimally safe environment, how to provide safe equipment to prevent falls, and describes the environmental features that facilitate patient mobility and safety.

ENSURING A SAFE ENVIRONMENT

Unfortunately, hospital units are not designed for patients; they do not enhance patient mobility or prevent falls. Rather, hospital environments are designed for the staff and for the ease of moving equipment, such as beds and wheelchairs. This is not to argue that it is impossible to improve environmental safety for a patient with a weak or impaired gait, but rather that funding will certainly help implementation of a safe environment.

THE WALKTHROUGH

The best way to assess the total environment is to plan a walk through with the Chief of Engineering, the Head of Housekeeping, the Vice President of Patient Care, the Director of Quality Assurance, and any other person involved in decision-making concerns in the hospital. As you enter each unit, the charge nurse for that particular unit could join the walkthrough, as his or her input is also important. If the hospital is planning an extension or renovation, it is important to involve the architects and other persons involved in planning.

STRUCTURAL FEATURES AS A THREAT TO PATIENT SAFETY

As previously stated, hospitals have been designed for the work of the staff rather than for patient safety. For instance, the patient's room has been designed to permit the gurney (or stretcher) to fit through the door and to be moved to either side of the bed so that the patient may be transferred safely. Unfortunately, hospital doorways are twice the width of domestic doorways. The bed may be placed in the center of the longest wall in the room, with no hand support for the patient to grasp when climbing out of bed. Often only the side rails (which are unsteady) and the bedside locker, which is on wheels, provide support for the patient. The patient's weakness and fatigue resulting from illness or surgery have been compounded by bed rest, so that from the patient's perspective it seems a very long and treacherous route to the bathroom. A serious concern is that often there are no additional handrails on the walls. Furthermore, should patients fall and hurt themselves on the furniture, the staff often paradoxically clear the room of all extraneous furniture, thereby removing the items that could be used for supportive handholds.

When patients with a weak or an impaired gait move about their rooms, they use the furniture for support and the position of the furniture determines the route they must take. When a gap in the supportive furniture occurs, the patient looks for the next support, takes several small steps, and "dives," arms outstretched, for the next support.

This "diving" is particularly dangerous for the elderly patient. Failing eyesight, diminishing coordination, and the extra distance that it takes to cross the room or reach the doorway results in what we call the "Wonderland phenomenon." This derives from the description of Alice's experiences in *Alice in Wonderland,* when everything appears larger as she becomes smaller. Spatial disorientation frequently occurs because the newly admitted patient has not yet learned the different dimension of the hospital environment, so that s/he often does not anticipate the differences when moving about. The distance from the bed to the bathroom may appear trivial to planners, but ask one of these people to lie on the bed. Ask them to consider how it must be to be 90 years of age, and now, try to get to the bathroom. Actually placing them in this position lets them see how the room must appear from the perspective of a patient.

Furthermore, although hospitals routinely place handrails in the hallways and in the bathroom, they are not installed in the patient's room—the area in which they are most needed! The solution to this problem is to create a safe path with supports for the patient to use between the bed and the bathroom.

Handrails

First, and most importantly, have handrails installed in the patients' rooms and on all walls between the bed and the bathroom.

Because this is the region where most falls occur and such rails may prevent or break a fall, thereby preventing injury, they are well worth the investment. Ideally, these rails should be rounded and installed out from the wall, providing the optimal grip using both the thumb and the fingers. Flat handrails, while serving the dual purpose of protecting the walls from damage with gurneys and other carts, force the patient to hold with a pinch grip, and this position of the hand is less effective than gripping a round rail. Handrails should be installed at an appropriate height, approximately 31 inches (.79 m or less) from the floor (Maki, Bartlett, & Fernie, 1985).

> Have handrails installed in the patient's rooms and on all walls between the bed and the bathroom.

Inspect the continuity of the rails, so that there will not be large gaps across doorways. Check that doors open in the direction that minimizes the distance that the patient has to walk to the bathroom. If the door hinges, for instance, are on the side of the patient's bed, the patient is then forced to walk around the door to get into the bathroom, increasing the distance that the patient must walk. Furthermore, large doors usually do not have anything other than the knob to hold on to.

There are special rails for installation around the toilet that will assist the patient in rising from the commode. So that these rails do not interfere with assisted transfer, they may be pushed against the wall when assistance is needed.

Often miscellaneous things, such as trays for charting or holding a computer, glove boxes, sharps boxes, hand sanitizer or masks, are fastened to the wall immediately above the handrails. These types of items interfere with the patient's safe use of the rail and are an impediment. Trays that are fixed to the wall present yet another problem. Because they prevent the installation of handrails, the patient may use the tray as a support, pulling it off the wall as they fall. Anticipate —and prevent—such incidents!!

Floors

Linoleum floors in the institution should be sealed with a matte, "nonglare" sealant (not polish). A shiny finish blinds elderly residents with poor visual accommodation. If the sun shines through windows and creates a glare (particularly down long corridors), then install blinds to block the sunshine. Many institutions are now using low pile carpets and, while these may provide better traction for walking, cleaning may be problematic. While carpeting provides more traction for the patient's feet when climbing out of bed, if the patient has an impaired gait and *slides* his or her feet along the floor when walking (i.e., the patient is not strong enough to lift his/her feet), then carpeting is likely to drag on the patient's slippers, thus contributing to a fall. Slippers with a smooth sole may, in part, relieve this problem, but those slippers then lack traction needed on tile and linoleum floors.

Be wary of dark decorative inlays in the flooring that may cause an additional hazard as a visual cliff. The sudden color change may startle the elderly patient and cause him to miss a step and fall.

Comfortable Seating

Because keeping elderly patients sitting upright in wheelchairs all day constitutes poor care, the unit must have safe comfortable seating for elderly patients. Recliners (with a waterproof seat cover) are ideal, as the patients may lie back and have their feet raised when they wish to rest. In addition, patients do not slide out of these chairs as easily as they tend to do from an upright chair. Hospital grade beanbag chairs are ideal for patients who are restless, making actual chair restraints (such as a Posey® belt or a gerichair with a locked tray) unnecessary. However, these chairs may also be considered a restraint, and patients placed in a beanbag chair must be observed carefully.

Safe Area for Wandering Patients

One of the reasons for the use of restraints is that many hospitals do not provide a supervised safe room for confused and wandering patients to walk. This safe area for wandering patients should be continuously supervised; it should contain comfortable chairs, a large space for "pacing," long areas with handrails on the walls for patients who need support when walking, a table for activities, large bright windows, and bathroom facilities.

Area, Bed, and Chair Alarms

If a separate area is not available for wandering patients or if the staff is afraid the patient will wander at night from his or her bedroom, a bed alarm, as well as an alarm system to alert nursing staff when a patient is leaving the area, may be a feasible option.

Area Alarms

Area alarms take two forms. The first consists of a sensor worn by the patient (usually around the ankle) and sensors installed in the doorways leading out of the unit. When the patient tries to leave the area, the sensor on the patient triggers the door alarm, thereby alerting staff, a member of which may then guide the patient back into the unit.

The second consists of alarms on the exit door that sound when the door is opened. While these alarms are excellent for home use, where they may be used to alert sleeping family members, in an institution they are most useful if installed on an individual patient's room door, so that the nurse may be alerted if the patient tries to leave the room.

Note that door alarms are only useful in preventing patients from wandering from the unit. Alternative methods exist for "securing" patients in an area where they may wander. The door to the area, for instance, could be fitted with two door handles approximately 12 inches apart (that the cognitively impaired would have difficulty opening) or the use of a "baffle latch" (Brungardt, 1994). Fabric strips may be placed across the door and fastened with Velcro to remind the wandering patient not to exit. Units must also consider other solutions, such as using volunteers or family members to sit with patients to discourage wandering behaviors.

Bed Alarms

Bed alarms are used to alert staff that a patient is getting out of bed. They should be used if the patient scores at high risk of falling. The nursing staff may then assist the patient in getting out of bed, getting up from a chair, or ambulating. Bed alarms provide an audible alarm when the patient moves toward the foot of the bed or tries to move out of the bed. Some beds have an alarm system installed in the bed itself; other alarms consist of a separate sensor that is placed under the patient's sheet at the level of the patient's buttocks and is connected to a sensor unit that is placed on the patient's side rails. The alarm may also be connected to the emergency or nurse call bell system.

The alarm sounds when the patient's weight is removed from the strip for a predetermined number of seconds, so that false alarms do not occur when the patient is turning in bed. The main disadvantage of these alarms is that if the patient is agile, the patient may be out of bed before the nurse arrives at the bedside to assist the patient.

Chair Alarms

Several types of chair alarms may be used to alert nursing staff when a patient attempts to get out of a chair. The first consists of disposable pressure sensitive strips that are placed on the seat of the chair and an alarm unit that is clipped on to the back of the chair. Once the patient has risen from the chair, the alarm sounds after a preset number of seconds. The second type is a connection between the patient and the alarm that sounds when the patient attempts to stand and becomes disconnected from the alarm.

When using chair alarms, these patients must be carefully observed. Since these alarms are activated when the patient stands (or attempts to stand), it is important that they not be used with patients who cannot bear weight.

Safe Beds

The patient's bed should be high-low adjustable, so that caregivers may raise the bed to provide care without incurring back injuries when lifting a patient. It should be an electric bed, with the controls for the backrest within the patient's reach. When the bed is in a low position, the *mattress* height (i.e., the height of the top surface of the mattress) should not be higher than a domestic bed (without the padded mattress top), so that when a patient of average height is sitting on the bed, both feet should be flat on the floor. The patient should neither have to "jump" to reach the floor when getting out of bed nor have to use a footstool.

When getting into bed, the patient should be able to manage this by sitting on the side of the bed, lying back while lifting the legs. Patients should never have to climb in to bed, as though climbing up a cliff! When the brake is on, the bed should not move at all—a person should be able to lean against the bed without it sliding, either by skidding on its brakes or slipping on the floor. Preferably, when the bed is in the low position, it should lock automatically. For transporting the patient, the ideal bed has wheels that "kick in" or the bed can be raised slightly off the floor. Finally, when moving, the wheels do not "shimmy"—they are steady, and the bed travels around corners easily.

Step Stools

Step stools are often provided to assist patients in climbing on to (or off of) a bed or an examination table. They may be necessary if the bed or examining table is unfortunately too high to otherwise reach, but caregivers must not forget that step stools are dangerous. The risk of injury is highest when the patient is climbing down from the bed and it is necessary to place both feet on the stool and then step on to the floor. Because of the risk of falling off the step stool, it is recommended that patients always have assistance when using the step stool.

Side Rails

The goal within any institution should be to reduce restraints, and it is important to remember that side rails are considered a restraint. Importantly, Capezuti, Wagner, Brush et al. (2007) found no relationship between reducing side rail use and bedside falls.

If the patient's bed is equipped with "split" side rails (i.e., 4 side rails, with two upper and two lower on each side), the lower rails should always be left down, to allow the patient a safe route from the bed. If all four rails are up, a confused patient may attempt to climb over the rails or over the end of the bed. Climbing over the rails increases the height that the patient may fall from and therefore increases the opportunity for serious injury; climbing over the end of the bed is a direct drop, or "cliff," which increases the impact of the fall, thereby increasing the chance for a serious injury. The use of full-length side rails (or having both upper and lower rails raised at the same time) is considered a restraint, as the patient does not have a safe route out of the bed. Because of the previously mentioned safety risks to the patient, these are not recommended.

> Side rails must not be used as a restraint.

The upper rails serve as a handhold to steady the patient when climbing into and out of bed by enabling the patient to sit up and pull on the rail, to turn, and to hang their legs over the side of the bed before standing. They also assist the patient when turning over by providing a firm rail to pull on as they turn or sit up. Top rails also remind the patient where the edge of the bed is and assist in preventing the patient from rolling or sliding out of bed.

If the patient's bed should be equipped with three-quarter length side rails, the patient has an exit route and may slide relatively safely from the bed, using the side rail as a handhold. Furthermore, the time required to "scoot" down to the end of the bed enables bed alarms time to sound a warning, thereby giving staff time to arrive to assist the patient. However, when the patient is getting into bed, three-quarter length side rails place the patient sitting on the end of the bed. The patient has some distance to "scoot" up in the bed to a correct position with his or her head on the pillow or must be lifted into position.

Call Bells

Call bells must be within easy reach of the patient, within easy reach of the commode and bathtubs, and answered promptly. When teaching patients to use a call bell, use the correct language. Some nurses tell patients to, "Be sure to *call* if you need anything." The nurses mean that patients should use the call bell, but patients remember only the instruction to *"call"* if they need anything, and lie back calling, "Nurse, Nurse"—and nobody can hear their feeble calling.

It should be noted that all call bells must be in excellent working order and checked periodically for necessary repairs.

Wheelchairs

Wheelchairs become safety hazards when they are poorly maintained. The foot rests should easily fold out of the patient's way when the patient tries to stand and not flop down and interfere with the patient's feet. The brakes must be easily applied, secured (i.e., hold the chair steady as the patient stands), and be easily released.

Wheelchairs tip under certain circumstances. For example, if the patient has his or her legs up and in plaster casts, then the chair is likely to become unbalanced and is prone to tip forward. Under these circumstances, the back of the wheelchair should be weighted to minimize the problem. If the patient deliberately leans back, the chair will fall backward, although there are anti-tip devices that may prevent these accidents, and these should be installed. The wheelchair can also tip sideways if the patient places his or her legs to the side while also moving his or her body weight to the same side. This becomes a risk when transferring the patient from the wheelchair to the bed.

Wheelchairs must be inspected regularly to ensure that they are kept in good repair. As wheelchairs come in various sizes, including large sizes for obese patients, and special sizes are not as readily available in the hospitals, nurses are sometimes reluctant to send them for repair as they cannot get a replacement to transport the patient in the interim. Other hospitals may use wheelchairs belonging to an outside transport company—and the wheelchairs belonging to the company have become mixed with their own stock. They continue to use these foreign chairs, but refuse to service them. In this way, their own patients are put at risk of an accident.

Chairs

Chairs for patients should not only be comfortable, but also safe. Often institutional concerns for hygiene result in vinyl covered chairs that are easy for the patient to slide out of. Chairs should have a wide seat, perhaps sloping slightly backward. They should also have a wide base for stability. When patients rise from a chair, they tend to push on the arms of the chair, causing the chair to sometimes slide backward. Chairs must be heavy enough to rise from without sliding, or they should be placed against a wall. The arms should be sturdy, as they are often used as a leverage to push against, when getting out of the chair.

IV Stands

Intravenous (IV) poles are often used by patients (particularly, postoperative patients) as walking aids. IV poles are not intended to be used as a walking aid, and unless they have an IV pump, they may be top heavy. Furthermore, when used as a walking aid, the patient must hold the IV pole out from their torso, so that their feet will not trip on the base, while watching that the top of the pole does not catch on a curtain rail or on the top of a doorway. Patients are also protective of the IV insertion site and may therefore hold that arm carefully against their bodies. Thus, the positions assumed when walking with an IV pole create another "accident about to happen." Compounding this issue is the fact that sometimes the wheels become clogged with dirt and dust, thereby sticking unexpectedly. When this happens, they roll unevenly and add an additional hazard for falling.

Canes, Walkers, and Crutches

Canes, walkers, and crutches must be inspected to ensure that the rubber tips are present and intact. Observe how they are used: Are they placed close to the patient, so they can be reached without a patient losing his/her balance? Are they used correctly when walking, or are they carried?

CONDUCTING EQUIPMENT SAFETY CHECKS

In hospitals, equipment that may place the patient "at risk" is checked on a regular basis by qualified staff. However, some equipment that is used daily, such as wheelchairs, may slip through the cracks and not be checked on a regular schedule. Most institutions appear to rely on the users and the nursing staff to request necessary repairs. Unfortunately, because most units do not have spare wheelchairs to replace those sent for repairs, necessary repairs are often postponed, and unsafe equipment remains in circulation.

> Check all equipment with maintenance personnel.

An equipment check on the unit should be undertaken initially by the maintenance person in charge of repairs. Start at one end of the unit and tag equipment that does not pass inspection with a sticker that includes the date. The major areas to be checked for safety are listed in Table 2.1.

It is important that the safety check be repeated at regular intervals, and the responsibility for conducting the survey should be assigned to a particular staff member. Checking equipment is not something that is simply done once and then forgotten.

Table 2.1

EQUIPMENT SAFETY CHECKLIST

Wheelchairs
Brakes	Secure chair when on?	_____
Arm rest	Detach easily for transfer bar?	_____
Leg rest	Easily adjusted?	_____
Foot pedals	Fold easily so that patient may stand?	_____
	Do not flop down?	_____
Wheels	Are not bent or warped?	_____
	Do not stick?	_____
	Anti-tip devices installed?	_____

IV Stands
Pole	Raises and lowers easily?	_____
Wheels	Roll easily and turn freely, do not stick?	_____
Stability	Will not tip over easily? (should be a 5-point base)	_____

Beds
Side rails	Raise and lower easily?	_____
	Secure when up?	_____
Wheels	Roll/turn easily, do not stick?	_____
Brakes	Secure bed when on?	_____

Footstools
Legs	Rubber skid protectors on feet?	_____
	Steady—does not rock?	_____
Top	Non-skid surface?	_____

Call Bells
Working?	Light outside door?	_____
	Buzzer sounds?	_____
	Alarms in nursing station?	_____
	Intercom satisfactory?	_____
	Accessible in bathrooms?	_____
	Cord pulls in good condition?	_____
	Room panel signals working?	_____

Walkers
Secure	Rubber tips present and in good condition?	_____
	Unit stable?	_____

Canes
Secure	Rubber tips in good condition?	_____

Crutches
Secure	Rubber tips in good condition?	_____

EQUIPMENT SAFETY CHECKLIST (*continued*)

Commodes
Wheels   Roll/turn easily, do not stick?   _____
            Are weighted and not "top heavy" when a
               patient is sitting on it?   _____

Gerichairs
If wheels   Roll/turn easily, do not stick?   _____
            Brakes secure when on?   _____
Tray   Secure?   _____

Handrails (Correct grip, as continuous as possible)
            In patient room   _____
            Bathroom   _____
            Hallways   _____

Walls   Glove boxes, chart trays, sharps boxes
            out of patients route to the bathroom?   _____

PATIENT SAFETY CARE PRACTICES

Ideally, nurses learn to routinely protect patients from hazardous situations, thereby preventing falls. For example, *placing the call bell within reach* is taught to nurses as a routine part of patient care from the first clinical experience. Nurses recognize that when reaching for a call bell, patients may lose balance and fall from the bed or a chair. Furthermore, a call bell that is out of reach is also "out of mind." Elderly

> The most frequently cited cause of falls is "going to the bathroom unassisted."

patients, in particular, may forget how to call the nurse, and when actual calling (i.e., shouting) fails to bring help, s/he may try to get out of bed unassisted, thereby risking a fall.

Similarly, personal belongings and things that are needed often, such as a water glass, should be within easy reach of the bed. Make sure that the patient's bedside stand is also within reach. Each time the nurse is with the patient, s/he should check that the patient has everything s/he needs.

The most frequently cited cause of falls is "going to the bathroom unassisted." Not only does this involve the risk of getting out of bed unassisted, but the patient, who is waiting for help to arrive, may also have waited until the last minute and is frequently in a hurry. Not only do urinary urgency and frequency add to the patient's haste, but if a patient is incontinent, a patient may slip in his/her urine. Good nursing care includes regular toileting of patients, especially at night. Patients should be routinely and regularly checked to see if they have any other needs and allowed to exercise or walk at least three times a day.

Safe, nonskid, well-fitting slippers are important. Patients often arrive in hospital with new, but impractical and unsafe, slippers. There may be scuffed or have slippery soles. Similarly, ill-fitting, disposable, hospital slippers made from foam are also impractical for walking—especially if the patient has an impaired gait—and should not be used.

Long bathrobes or female patients' long nightgowns that reach the floor are very dangerous as the patient may tread on the hem and fall. This hazard may become more problematic if the patient has had abdominal surgery and walks with a stooped gait, attempting to protect the wound and prevent pain. Hospital gowns that open at the back and are secured with two or three ties also create a fall risk because the patient may lose his/her balance when walking, attempting to preserve modesty by holding the gown closed in back. The best solution is to give the patient two gowns to wear, one over the other, with one tied at the back and one tied at the front.

The night lighting must be bright enough for the patients to become quickly oriented on waking and to remember where they are. Night lighting must be bright enough for patients to find their bedside lighting and call bells, to find their slippers and gowns, to find their way safely to the bathroom without falling over or walking into anything, and to find the bathroom light switches. Nightlights that provide a reasonable glow and are set close to the floor are a good solution: bright lights that shine into a room from a bathroom or hallway may be so bright as to interfere with sleep or temporarily blind the patient on waking. Finally, it is important to have a clear policy for whomever is responsible for immediately wiping up spills on to the floor, and for signposting wet and slippery areas.

REFERENCES

Brungardt, G. S. (1994). Patient restraints: New guidelines for a less restrictive approach. *Geriatrics, 49*(6), 43–50.

Capezuti, E., Wagner, L., Brush, B., Boltz, M., Renz, S., & Talerico, K. (2007). Consequences of an intervention to reduce restrictive side rail use in nursing homes. *The American Geriatrics Society, 55,* 334–341.

Maki, B. E., Bartlett, S. A., & Fernie, G. R. (1985). Effect of stairway pitch on optimal handrail height. *Human Factors, 27*(3), 355–350.

REFERENCES

3 Monitoring Falls in the Institution

Monitoring falls, the injuries resulting from falls, and the eventual outcome of a fall are all crucial. This chapter considers not just monitoring the ramifications of a fall, but also how to evaluate the success of your fall intervention program. Monitoring provides the means to inform the nurses and the administration of the seriousness of the problem of falls and the effectiveness of fall intervention strategies. Regular reporting of the fall rates of each unit, as well as the total institution, motivates the staff to continue fall prevention efforts, as it provides them with the satisfaction of observing the incidence of falls—and of serious injuries—decline.

RECORDING FALL RATES

Defining a Fall

Unfortunately, a satisfactory definition of a hospital fall does not exist. In 1980, Morris and Isaacs defined it as an event in which "the patient came to rest on the floor." This broad definition, however, is flawed. For example, it includes patients who slipped from a chair onto the floor, patients who were found lying on the floor but were not actually seen falling, and falls in which a bystander caught the patient (thereby reducing the impact of the fall) but in which the patient was lowered to the floor. It does not, however, include patients who have fallen, but managed to flop down onto a bed or into a chair, rather than land on the floor, or patients who fell and were not found, but managed to get up unassisted. Finally, it does not include a slip in a bathtub or many other possible occurrences. Thus, although in some instances it is very clear when a patient falls or has fallen, other instances leave room for interpretation. Compounding the problem is the fact that patients who are fall prone are very often poor historians regarding an actual fall. They may not consider a slip or a trip a *real* fall; they may forget to report that they fell, or they may be too embarrassed to mention the event to a staff member.

Exactly what constitutes a fall is, therefore, left to the best judgment of the staff member. However, it is important to note that if the fall prevention program is going to reduce falls, the goal is to prevent all falls, *including the first fall.* Therefore, if a staff member *prevents* a fall by catching a patient, for instance, then this should be noted in the patient's record. A "missed fall" is a useful piece of information for improving a fall prevention strategy.

It is important that falls reported in the fall database be only *patient* falls. If a staff member or a visitor falls, it must be reported and recorded somewhere else, otherwise the database will be inflated with incidents other than *patient* falls. Furthermore, a patient must have *fallen,* not been *dropped* by a staff member, to be recorded in the patient falls database.

Falls count as a *fall* if the person was trying to get out of bed to walk when the fall occurred or if the patient was being transferred from a wheelchair to a bed or a gurney. It is important to note that the instruments for identifying fall-proneness assume that the person will experience a fall while walking. Therefore, the database should not include falls by toddlers who fell, for instance, while climbing onto the back of a chair.

How to Measure the Incidence of Falls in the Institution

A number of methods can be used to measure the incidence of falls in an institution, and these methods are not equivalent. It is recommended that institutions select and report their incidence of falls using the *Fall Rate*. The *Fall Rate* is the most reliable, because it includes *all falls* in its calculation, not just the number of patients *who have fallen*. While a patient who falls repeatedly may apparently artificially inflate the statistics, it is an accurate reflection of the number of times a patient is actually at risk of injury. The *Fall Rate* also is calculated using the number of *patient bed days*, rather than the number of patients at risk, which does not consider the length of stay.

The *Fall Rate* is be calculated using the following formula:

$$\frac{\text{number of patient falls}}{\text{number of patients bed days}} \times 1,000$$

However, because the formula is not restricted to a particular time frame, it is important to state the period for which the statistics were collected for future reference. Therefore your fall rate should state the period (i.e., for a 12-month period).

When starting to measure the fall rate, note one warning: The initiation of a fall prevention program often results in a change of attitude among staff members. Previously, it may have been a nuisance to complete a fall report form or it may have been considered an indicator of poor care and a reason for self-blame. A prevention program, however, suddenly makes it acceptable to have a resident fall. The attitude shifts from "Why did *I* let this patient fall?" to "Why didn't this strategy work?" This removal of personal responsibility from the incident results in an increase in reporting of resident falls. This, in turn, results in an apparent change in the fall rate. Just when the fall rate should be decreasing, the change in reporting falls results in an apparent increase in the fall rate.

To calculate the patient fall rate, suppose an institution collected the following statistics:

Number of patient falls (2006 calendar year)   147

Number of patient bed days (2006 calendar year)   49,946

Using these data, the fall rate for the institution may be as follows:

$$\frac{147}{49,946} \times 1,000 = 2.9 \text{ per } 1,000 \text{ patient bed days for 2006.}$$

However, not all institutions (or authors of research articles, for that matter) use this statistic. Other institutions may report such statistics as *the number of patients at risk, the number of patients who fell, the number of falls per bed,* or *the probability of falling.* Appendix C compares methods for calculating fall rates.

THE INJURY RATE

If you believe that whether or not a patient is injured when s/he falls is strictly a matter of chance, then you see no relationship between the fall rate and the injury rate—it would be random. But this is not the case, and institutions will find that there is often some consistency between the two statistics. But that is not why the injury rate is important; the injury rate is important because it is the bottom line. We may not be able to prevent all types of falls, or even all falls—especially if we are encouraging ambulation, but it is our responsibility to lower our injury rate as much as possible. This is your most important statistic.

In addition, the injury rate is a more reliable statistic than the fall rate, because staff members are careful to complete an incident report form when an injury occurs. Since it is really the *injuries* that are problematic, the injury rate provides an important indicator in monitoring institutional falls.

The injury rate percentage for any time period may be calculated as follows:

$$\frac{\text{number of patients injured}}{\text{number of patients who fell}} \times 100$$

To avoid artificially inflating the statistic, be sure to enter each patient fall in the database once, even if the patient received more than one injury. For instance, if a patient fractured an arm and a hip in the same fall, count that as *one* patient who was injured. In addition, when demonstrating the efficacy of a fall prevention program, it may be helpful for the institution to calculate the rate of *minor, moderate,* and *major* injuries separately. For example, a trial to test the efficacy of the *Morse Fall Scale (MFS)* at the Veterans Affairs Medical Center in Portland, Oregon (see, McCollam, 1995) showed that the fall rate increased 24% (perhaps as a result of changes in reporting norms and including near-falls in the calculation), but the number of serious injuries from falls *fell* 174% to an all time low of four falls. However, the injury rate was not reported.

CLASSIFYING INJURIES

Classifying the degree of injury is important for purposes of analysis. Although it is relatively easy to classify injuries into two or three categories (usually minor and serious or minor, moderate, and major), it is important that the criteria for classification are published so that others may compare their data.

At present, there is a confusing array of classifications. Some authors have only included fractures in the "major" category, while others have included incidences of head injuries (such as a concussion), soft tissue injury requiring suturing, and fractures. It is recommended that the classification system shown in Table 3.1 be used when classifying the seriousness of an injury.

A second problem that may occur when using the injury rate is that often injuries are not diagnosed for several days after the incident. For instance, after an elderly patient falls, a minor injury, such as a bruised hip, may be reported. However, if the patient continues to complain of pain several days after the incident, an x-ray will be ordered and a hairline fracture of the pelvis may be diagnosed at that time. In these cases, it is important to

Use a standardized method of classifying injury.

Table 3.1

CLASSIFICATION OF SEVERITY OF INJURY

No Injury: No evidence of abrasion or bruising and no complaint of pain following the fall.

Minor: Any small bruise or abrasion that does not require medical treatment and will heal within several days.

Moderate: Injury requiring medical treatment that is not considered major. For example, a small cut that requires only a few sutures, or an IV that infiltrates and needs to be reinserted. Bruises and contusions are considered moderate if they require treatment, and sprains, as well as suspected bone injury are considered moderate if an X-ray is ordered and there is no fracture.

Major: A serious injury including any fracture, head injury, or wound that requires major suturing.

correct the original fall report form. Thus, quality assurance personnel must routinely follow-up on patient falls and injuries approximately 4 days after the fall. Furthermore, patients who have been seriously injured must be monitored until the consequences and outcome of their falls and injuries are known. In many instances, the eventual outcome of a fractured hip in an elderly patient is death from pneumonia weeks or several months after the incident. These outcomes, however, are usually not included in the incident report form nor are they noted by the administration.

> Routinely follow-up with patients 4 days after the initial fall to ensure that injuries were not subsequently diagnosed.

COMMON ERRORS IN REPORTING

Because a number of methods are used to report patient falls, it is often difficult to compare the fall rate between institutions, between patient populations, and/or when evaluating fall prevention programs.

Often the length of time for which data were collected is not reported. Readers are also frequently unable to ascertain if one patient has fallen many times (which are dependent events), and whether this information has been included in the calculations.

Because there are difficulties with some of the methods used, it is recommended that the fall rate (i.e., the number of falls/number of patient bed days x 1,000) be used as the standard measure. Other statistics, such as the number of patients at risk, the number of repeated falls, and the number of patients injured, can be reported, so that all necessary calculations and comparisons can be made, but the fall rate should be the standard statistic used when benchmarking. And finally, if, after implementing a fall prevention program, the expected reduction in fall rate does not occur, administrators should examine all possible reasons for failure, including changes in staffing levels, patient acuity, and reporting norms. Remember that the most important statistic is *injury rate.*

> To reduce error, use the *fall rate* as the standard measure.

ESTABLISHING BASELINE DATA

In The United States, a fall intervention program is no longer optional. Rather, it is an essential component for accreditation. All institutions must also evaluate how serious the problem of patient falls is in their institution compared to others with similar patient populations. Thus, the first step is to use available data from hospital statistics and create a table or bar graph to illustrate the incidence of falls covering as many years as possible. Examine the fall rate and the injury rate for each year. Compare these rates. Were they consistent over the years? From these statistics, it will be possible to ascertain how serious the problem of patient falls is in the institution. After implementing a fall intervention program, these statistics will provide the evidence necessary to show the reduction of the fall rate and the injury rate, further justifying the cost of the fall intervention program.

INSTITUTIONAL MONITORING

Deciding What to Count

Chapter 1 discussed the ambiguity of defining a fall exactly. When a patient falls, it is often clear that the patient has fallen because the nurse may observe the fall or hear the thud as the patient hits the floor. But if a patient slips and prevents him or herself from falling by grabbing the handrail, does that "almost-a-fall" count as a fall, and should an incident form be completed? Similarly, if a patient is at the end of the bed and found (and caught) by a nurse as he or she is about to fall, that is a prevented fall—*a near miss*—a successfully prevented fall. Since the actual fall did not occur, how is that incident communicated to other staff?

When deciding on the efficacy of a program, the administration needs to decide if in addition to counting actual falls, it will count the "near misses"—the prevented falls—as an additional indicator of the program's success. Prevented falls could be listed separately and noted by the unit. Not only are they a means to provide credit to the nurses who prevented the incident, but they provide additional data about the patient's fall risk; the time, the place, and the context of possible falls; and possible future reoccurrence.

How to Record a Fall

Staff members routinely record information about a fall on an *Incident Report Form*. These forms request information about the patient's activity and the events surrounding the fall, including witnesses, date and time of fall, how many previous falls the patient has had, any injury and treatments required, and whether family and physicians were notified of the fall. There should also be space to list the patient's *MFS*—the scores for each item and the total score before the fall. These forms become part of the permanent record in the patient's chart and are also reviewed by the Risk Management team and the Fall Clinical Nurse Specialist. The Fall Clinical Nurse Specialist then conducts a fall assessment and schedules a conference about the patient with the multidisciplinary team. As a fall is highly likely to reoccur, the fall needs to be communicated to all of the staff members who will care for the patient throughout the hospital stay.

Some institutions do this through a *Fall Log Record,* which lists each patient who falls, where the fall occurred, the patient activity at the time of the fall, and the time the fall occurred. Each patient should be listed in a separate section, because if a subsequent fall occurs, as mentioned in Chapter 6, the *Fall Log Record* will aid in identifying patterns of falls and help reduce the recurrence of falls.

Whose Responsibility Is It to Monitor Falls?

The primary responsibility for monitoring patient falls belongs to the Fall Clinical Nurse Specialist. In many institutions, it is his/her responsibility to collate the fall statistics, coordinate the fall consultation team, provide feedback to the patient's primary nurse, and ensure that all shifts are aware of the special fall prevention strategies developed for certain patients. The Fall Clinical Nurse Specialist must prepare monthly reports on the number of falls and the number and type of injuries, both for each unit and the institution as a whole. These reports should also show the statistics for the previous month and for the same period the previous year. This feedback to staff is vital because it aids in demonstrating that their prevention efforts are worthwhile. However, recall that the fall rate will increase over the period just prior to the initiation of the program because of changes in reporting norms.

REFERENCES

McCollam, M. (1995). Evaluation and implementation of a research-based falls assessment innovation. *Nursing Clinics of North America, 30*(3), 507–514.

Morris, E. V., & Isaacs, B. (1980). The prevention of falls in a geriatric hospital. *Age and Ageing, 9,* 1981–1985.

4 Predicting Physiological Anticipated Falls

The nursing approach is based on the underlying assumption that falls should not occur if the care is excellent. This places considerable responsibility on the individual staff member as well as the institution. For example, Arsenault (1982) writes:

"It could have happened to any of us!" These words keep reverberating in my head as I remember my return to work after an eight day vacation.

It was a calm Saturday evening. Mr. Smith was one of my five patients. He was an elderly man admitted to the hospital for treatment of an aspirate pneumonia. He was physically improving, but he continued to have diarrhea secondary to Iscal tube feedings. To prevent fecal incontinence, Mr. Smith routinely used his commode unattended before he retired to bed. So I left him on his commode [while I left] to care for another patient. This evening, Mr. Smith never did make it back to bed. Five minutes later I was summoned to his room . . . There he lay—ashen, unresponsive and bleeding from a gash in his head. He had fallen while attempting to walk to the bathroom. Mr. Smith died two weeks later. (p. 386)

Thus, even if the fall was primarily caused by the patient's underlying medical condition, nurses apparently feel that it is their responsibility to *prevent any fall from occurring.*

ASSESSING FALL RISK: PATIENT ASSESSMENT

Because of the diverse perspectives on the reasons underlying patient falls, there are basically three types of instruments (scales) available to assist in identifying the patient who falls. The first group consists of scales that separate the patients who may fall from those who may not; these also *predict the likelihood* of a patient falling. In this way, fall prevention strategies and resources may be targeted to *prevent* falls in the patients most likely to fall. These forms are short, quick, and easy to use. The patient's fall risk is not stable, but rather changes throughout the day. These forms are intended to be used frequently— at least once daily.

The second group, *fall assessment forms,* assist staff in identifying the possible causes of falls. These forms usually include some environmental checks (such as bed in the low position), patient behaviors (patient gait, confusion), nursing care strategies (toilet patient regularly, remind patient to use call bell), possible problems in the medical regimen (number of medications), and prevention strategies (reinforce fall risk with families). These long and cumbersome forms are intended to be used once, usually on admission.

The third type is designed to be used *after the patient has fallen.* These forms consist of a space to write details of the fall itself, including the patient's account of the incident, patient behavior at the time the incident occurred, any injures sustained, a physical examination checklist to record the patient's condition, and any recommendation for prevention in the future. These forms are also long and cumbersome.

As already mentioned, when selecting a method of assessing patient falls it is important that the instrument is used as intended and published by the researcher who developed it. Changing any of the items or the item scores destroys the reliability and validity of the *Scale* and thus its ability to predict falls. Similarly, while it is tempting to "improve" these scales by creating your own—for instance, by selecting the apparent "best" items from several scales, such measures may result in a scale with no reliability or validity. Select a scale that has reported reliability and validity, and use it in its entirety.

THE *MORSE FALL SCALE*

The *Morse Fall Scale* (MFS) is a rapid and simple method of assessing a patient's likelihood of falling. It consists of six variables that are quick and easy to score, and it has been shown to have predictive validity and interrater reliability.[1]

Method of *Scale* Construction

Patients who fell (*n*=100) and 100 randomly selected controls were examined using a comprehensive physical examination form, inspection of contributing environmental factors, the patient's report of the fall, and the outcome (including patient injuries). Significant variables that differentiated the patients who fell from the patients who did not fall were identified using techniques of discriminant analysis and data reduction. *Scale* weights were obtained for each significant variable (item) and, using techniques of computer modeling, the *Scale* was tested on a simulated patient population. Validity was further established by randomly splitting the data set and repeating the procedures used to obtain the significant variables, and then testing them on the remaining 50% of these data (See Appendix A).

Examination of False Negatives

The charts of 22 patients who had fallen and who were not classified as fall-prone by the *MFS* were examined. This analysis showed that all

---

[1] *Reliability and Validity:* Interrater reliability scores on the *Scale* using 21 raters, was $R = 0.96$. To obtain consistency, videotapes of patient's ambulating were used for this trial (Morse et al., 1989). A test for internal consistency revealed poor interitem correlation, with a coefficient alpha of .16. This, combined with the results of analysis of variance ($f = 71.34$, $p < .00001$), suggest that the *Scale* items are relatively independent (see Appendix B).

patients were oriented. Despite the fact that eight patients had a weak gait, only one used a walking aid. These patient falls were classified as *"unanticipated physiological falls."*

Prospective Testing

Sixteen patient care units, from three types of patient care areas.(i.e., acute medical and surgical, long-term geriatric care, and rehabilitation areas) from two institutions used the *MFS* for a 4-month period. Daily rating of all patients resulted in 2,689 patients examined for fall score and a subsequent fall. Examination of scores in the acute care institution by length of stay revealed different patterns of fall risk; the mean score of the long-term patients showed less variation and higher scores. Analysis of patients who fell by type of fall (anticipated, unanticipated, and accidental) and the severity of injuries increased with the higher scores, indicating clinical validity of the *Scale* (see Appendix B).

SCORING THE *MORSE FALL SCALE*

Testing in the clinical area by nurses who used the *Scale* as a part of their normal work day showed that the *MFS* is quick and easy to use. Of the nurses, 82.9% rated the *Scale* as "quick and easy to use," while 54% estimated that it took less than 3 minutes to rate a patient.

The items in the *Scale* (see Table 4.1) are scored as indicated in the following subsections.

History of Falling

This is scored as 25 if the patient has fallen during the present hospital admission or if there was an immediate history of physiological falls. Examples include falls from seizures or an impaired gait prior to admission. If the patient has not fallen, history of falling is scored 0. **NOTE:** If a patient falls for the first time, then his/her score immediately increases by 25.

Table 4.1

MORSE FALL SCALE			
ITEM			**SCORE**
1. History of Falling	no	0	
	yes	25	____
2. Secondary Diagnosis	no	0	
	yes	15	____
3. Ambulatory Aid			
none/bed rest/nurse assist		0	
crutches/cane/walker		15	
furniture		30	____
4. Intravenous Therapy/Saline Lock	no	0	
	yes	20	____
5. Gait			
normal/bed rest/wheelchair		0	
weak		10	
impaired		20	____
6. Mental Status			
oriented to own ability		0	
overestimates/forgets limitations		15	____
		Total	____

Secondary Diagnosis

This is scored as 15 if more than one medical diagnosis is listed on the patient's chart; if not, the score is 0.

Ambulatory Aids

This is scored as 0 if the patient walks without a walking aid (even if assisted by a nurse), uses a wheelchair, or is on bed rest and does not get out of bed at all. If the patient uses crutches, a cane, or a walker, this item scores 15; if the patient ambulates clutching on to the furniture for support, score this item 30.

Intravenous Therapy

This is scored as 20 if the patient has an intravenous apparatus or a saline lock inserted; if not, score 0.

Gait

The characteristics of the three types of gait are evident regardless of the type of physical disability, or underlying cause. A normal gait is characterized by the patient walking with head erect, arms swinging freely at the side, and striding unhesitantly. This gait scores 0.

With a *weak gait* (scored as 10), the patient is stooped but is able to lift his/her head while walking without losing balance. If support from furniture is required, this is with a featherweight touch for reassurance, rather than a grabbing to remain upright.

With an *impaired gait* (scored as 20), the patient may have difficulty rising from a chair, attempting to get up by pushing on the arms of the chair and/or by "bouncing" (i.e., by using several attempts to rise). The patient's head is down, and s/he focuses on the ground. Because the patient's balance is poor, the patient grasps on to the furniture, a support person, or a walking aid, and cannot walk without this assistance. When assisting the patient to walk, the nurse will note that s/he *really* holds on to the nurse's hand. When grasping a rail or furniture, the patient holds so tightly that his/her knuckles turn white. The patient takes short steps and shuffles.

If the patient is in a wheelchair, the patient is scored according to the gait s/he used when transferring from the wheelchair to the bed. Steps are short, and the patient may shuffle.

Dear Jan,

Does the *MFS* work with a neuro population who experience impulsivity and impaired balance?

Sincerely,
Judy

Dear Judy,

Score "impulsivity" in mental status;
Score "impaired balance" in gait.

Jan

Mental Status

When using the *Scale,* mental status is measured by checking the patient's own self-assessment of his or her ability to ambulate. Ask the patient, "Are you able to go to the bathroom alone, or do you need assistance?" If the patient's reply in judging his/her own ability is consistent with the ambulatory orders on the nurse's orders, the patient is rated as "normal" and scored 0. If the patient's response is not consistent with the nursing orders, or if the patient's assessment is unrealistic, then the patient is considered to be *overestimating his/her abilities* and to be *forgetful of limitations.* Score this as 15.

Final Score

The score is then tallied and recorded on the patient's chart.

It is important that none of the items on the *Scale* are omitted or changed. For example, some long-term care institutions may not use IV therapy. If this is the case, *leave IV therapy on the Scale*—it will simply always be zero for that institution. It is also important ***not*** *to simplify the scores, for instance, by changing the values to single digits, as this will result in the loss of validity.* For example, changing the score to 1s and 0s results in a loss of almost 30% of the number of falls correctly identified and gives a scale that predicts a fall-prone patient only slightly better than by chance. To assist nurses to remember the items and scoring system, it is recommended to make a small pocket card version of the *Scale* available to the staff.

Dear Jan,

The *MFS* has nothing about medications. Can I add that item?

Julie

_____

Hi Julie,

Medications are a part of the *Scale*; they are included in the comorbidity/secondary diagnosis score.

When developing the indices (items), we first included medications that were thought to contribute to falls (this was not significant) and then the numbers of medications (this was significant). We then combined this last item with comorbidity (secondary Dx). This means patients who have more that one presenting complaint receive more than one set of medications, and it is this polypharmacy that contributes to their fall risk.

Of course, medications contribute to fall risk as they relate to the other variables (mainly gait and mental status). This means that if there is a serious problem with medications, they will contribute to the *MFS* score in those categories.

I recommend that if a patient score is high risk for falling, then a patient assessment should be conducted. It should include a review of medications, with the goal of reducing the medications or side effects, thereby reducing the patient's fall score.

One last thing, NEVER add or alter a *MFS* item or assigned score, as this will interfere with the validity of the *Scale*. You do not have permission to alter the copyrighted *MFS*.

Jan

Hi Jan,

The item values are clumsy—why are they not 1s, 2s, and 3s?

Janette

Dear Janette,

The *MFS* works because the items selected were statistically significant and because these values are weighted according to their contribution to falls. In other words, if we changed these scores (and made the numbers easier to add), then the *MFS* would lose or seriously impair its ability to determine who is likely to fall.

Jan

DETERMINING LEVEL OF RISK

The risk of falling varies greatly with different patient populations, as well as at different times of day and different stages of the patient's illness. Therefore, ideally, the *MFS* should be *calibrated to each unit*, so that fall prevention strategies are targeted to those most at risk (within the range of 25 to 55).

This is important: Institutionwide, in an acute care hospital, the *Scale* could be set with a high risk cut-off score of 25. This is because in an acute care hospital, there are many patients with a normal gait, who are not at risk of falling. However, those who are at highest risk are "clustered" on certain units (such as the psychogeriatric unit). If a cut-off score for high risk was set at 25 on those units, then all of the patients would score at high risk. (Of course, in some units *all* of the patients may be at very high risk of falling, and fall prevention measures should be provided for all those patients.) Thus, the high-risk score should vary according to the type of patients on the unit, but should never be higher than 55. If a units consists of all high-risk patients, such as stroke patients, the *Scale* should be set at about 45, with all patients targeted for fall prevention strategies. On a surgical unit, only a few of the patients will be at very high risk of falling, and the *Scale* should be set at about 25.

> Calibrate the *MFS* for each particular unit, so that fall prevention strategies are targeted to those most at risk.

Hi Jan,

There is a note in the book that the *MFS* has to be calibrated for each clinical area. Can you tell me more about this?

Liz

_____

Hi Liz,

Calibrating or determining the "cut off" score to determine high risk can be established by administrators for each area. Alternatively, administrators may decide to use one score to indicate high risk for all areas. If you choose the latter, do not set the *Scale* higher than 45.

The higher you set the *Scale,* the fewer patients you have scoring "at risk." This does not mean that their actual risk of falling changes, but it does mean that you will not be providing those at risk with fall protective strategies. Conversely, if you set the scale too low, your "at-risk" population will grow to include many patients at varying levels of risk, thereby decreasing *Scale* sensitivity.

Jan

Deciding on the high risk score is very important because if the cut-off score from a unit with many disabled patients is applied generally throughout the hospital, the cut-off score will be set too high. The *Scale* will lose its sensitivity, and many of the patients who are at risk of falling will not be protected (i.e., the false negative rate will increase).[2] The highest cut-off scores that Morse has set on the *Scale* is 45, which was in a rehabilitation hospital and a nursing home. In this case, a "medium risk group" was also established with scores between 35 and 44.

On no account should the high risk score be set above 55.

There are several ways to determine the cut-off score to be used. The best method is to score all the patients in a unit and examine the distribution of these scores. In consultation with administration, the CNS should determine the cut-off score for the percentage of patients that will be declared "high risk," along with considering the costs of providing a fall prevention program and the benefits of the program.

---

[2] In an early trial of the *Scale* at the Veterans Affairs Medical Center in Portland, Oregon, a cut-off score of 55 was determined efficient from a pilot study in a cardiology general-medical unit. This was extremely high and resulted in the loss of sensitivity of the *Scale*. The authors concluded that "As suggested by Morse, cut-off scores need to be adjusted for different patient groups" (McCollam, 1995, p. 514). This is not exactly correct.

Examine the distribution of the scores with the scores obtained in Morse's study (Table B.1 and Table D.2) to see if the distribution of scores obtained in your institution for a particular unit are similar. Examine Table D.2 to see the number of fall-prone patients who would be missed (considered false negatives), or the number of patients *not* at risk who are scored "at risk" (considered false positives) and receive fall prevention for various level of the *Scale*. Consultation with the hospital administration may be necessary at this time, because the level of high risk set for the unit has cost implications in providing fall prevention measures. There may also be legal implications if a patient falls or is injured, and there is a subsequent lawsuit against the hospital.

USING THE *MORSE FALL SCORE*

Score Frequently

Patients' risk scores should be evaluated at least once per shift in order to monitor fall risk adequately. In long-term care, where patients fall risks are more stable, the patients should be scored frequently over several 24-hour periods, until their fall risk pattern is recognized. After that, less frequent scoring—even once a week is adequate—if the resident's condition does not change.

A major problem is not scoring the patient frequently enough. For instance, a standard has emerged that patients are scored on admission and if the patients' conditions change. Scoring just twice is not frequently enough for patients in acute care, where fall risk changes rapidly.

Record the Patient's Score as Well as the Level of Risk

When using the *MFS*, always be aware of the patient's actual score. Because the *MFS* is sensitive to changes in the patient's fall risk, you can use the scale score to determine an improvement or decline in the patient's condition. Just as a patient's temperature would lose meaning if you recorded only "normal" and "high," so does the patient's fall risk if you consider it only as "low," "medium," and high."

Correct Assessment

If the scale is going to perform accurately, staff must learn how to use the *Scale* correctly. The *MFS* consists of items that must be scored both from the patient's chart and from direct patient assessment. When the *Scale* was first developed, an instructional videotape was available to teach the use of the *Scale*. In 2003, this was replaced with an instructional CD, provided for a small charge from Hill Rom Industries.[3] Many hospitals have put the CD-Rom on their computing system, so that the training program may be readily accessed by staff. Some have even negotiated with the State Board of nursing for CEUs for those who have completed the training. Despite the availability of these instructional tools, some do not realize that scoring the patient **requires that the patient be examined.** Hospitals using the *Scale* must provide in-service education for nurses regarding the use of the *Scale*. As with all forms of assessment, if the scale is not used correctly, regardless of the reliability and validity of the *Scale*, it is of no use in the clinical area.

Recognize the Sensitivity of the *Scale*

The staff must record the patient's actual total score, as well as the high-risk or low-risk score. Again, think of this as recording a patient's temperature, rather than just "a high temperature." If the actual temperature is not recorded, the staff will not know if the temperature is increasing or decreasing, or be able to determine the severity of the fever. Similarly if the staff does not record the actual fall score, then the staff members will not know how high the fall risk is. Furthermore, the goal of care is to lower the score, and if the actual score is not recorded—or the values for each time—then it will not be possible to note improvement (and decrease of risk) or an increasing score (and therefore increased risk) of falling.

---

[3] CD ROM order # CTG581 Pocket cards of the MFS are also available. Online http://www.hill-rom.com/usa/PS_Nofalls.htm (click the "Preventing Patient Falls" button)

Finally, a frequent complaint from the clinical areas is that all of the patients scored high risk of falling. It is possible that all of the patients are, for instance, at high risk. Raising the level of risk will not change this fact, but it will place those who are at risk in the "not-at-risk" category. But if the actual score is recorded, then the staff will recognize that there are degrees of high risk.

Dear Mrs. Morse,

We have seen some people use a high risk cut off of 51 or greater. Do you still recommend keeping 45 as the cut off?

Sincerely,
Jenny

Dear Jenny,

Yes.

Best wishes,
Jan

PREPARING TO IMPLEMENT A FALL PREVENTION PROGRAM

Once the administrative decision has been made to invest in a fall prevention program, the structures necessary for the program must be put in place. These structures consist of appointing a clinical nurse specialist to be responsible for the implementation of the program (including providing inservice to staff) and the setting up of an interdisciplinary consultation team.

The Role of the Clinical Nurse Specialist

A clinical nurse specialist should be appointed as *fall prevention nurse* in the institution. This nurse will be responsible for setting up a recording system for reporting falls, ensuring that all staff members are able to use the *MFS* reliably through inservice education, conducting fall assessment of high risk patients, and establishing fall protection regimes, conducting multidisciplinary team meetings regarding very high risk patients and patients who fall repeatedly, providing staff with inservice education of fall prevention strategies, and meeting with relatives regarding the use of (or decisions not to use) restraints. The nurse will conduct fall assessment on high risk patients and consult with physical therapists, occupational therapists, and physicians. The nurse will do follow-up on all patients who have fallen, identify fall prevention strategies, prepare care plans accordingly, and make recommendations to prevent reoccurrence. S/he will track all patients who are injured in a fall to determine the impact of the injury on the patient's subsequent health and mobility levels. The fall prevention nurse specialist is also responsible for conducting (with maintenance staff) environmental and equipment safety checks of all units on a regular basis. Finally, s/he is responsible for the regular calculation of fall and injury rates and the reporting of these to staff and administration on a regular basis.

> A clinical nurse specialist leads the fall prevention program.

Teaching Staff

Inservice instruction of all staff regarding the use of the *MFS* appears a formidable task, but is not so onerous if conducted in small group sessions. Once the initial instruction is complete, with the incorporation of the module into the regular staff orientation program, the use of the *Scale* becomes a routine and simple task. In McCollam's study, the staff reported that the *Scale* took only 1 minute to complete and recommended that it become a part of the regular assessment forms.

A Web site sponsored by Hill Rom safety program on the use of the *Scale* is available http://www.hill-rom.com/usa/Safety_PatientFalls.htm. This program takes 10 minutes to view. It is also recommended that the *Scale* be reproduced on cards that staff members can carry around in their pockets. They are then prepared to refer frequently to the items on the *Scale* and their values.

Even if the decision has been made to score patients regularly once a day, it is important that all staff, even night staff, be familiar with and able to use the *MFS*.

This is because of the variability of patients' fall risks should their conditions change. For instance, patients may *only* be confused at night (as with "sundowners"), and their judgment regarding their ability to go into the washroom unassisted at night is impaired. In such cases, the score for mental status of these patients would increase by 15 points at night, and this should be documented on the patient's chart. Alternatively, nurses may find that patients are more tired when they are assisting patients back to bed, and their gait changes from weak to impaired, and their fall score increases accordingly. In this way, patients' fall scores may fluctuate in a 24-hour period, and the staff should be sensitive to such variability.

> All staff must be familiar with and be able to use the *MFS*.

Hello Jan,

I am in the process of implementing a fall risk assessment and prevention program at our hospital. I am using your fall scale for our inpatient population, but have problems applying it to the outpatient areas. Our outpatient areas include a busy emergency department, radiology, cardiology, and behavioral health unit. Can you recommend a fall risk assessment for these areas?

Be good,
Cynthia

_____

Hi Cynthia,

In Emergency Departments, I recommend that the staff only score patients who are at obvious risk of anticipated falls. Triage by asking 3 questions:

1. Has the patient fallen before (or is the patient in ED as a result of a fall)?
2. Does the patient have an impaired gait?
3. Is the patient cognitively impaired?

Use the *MFS* asap if any of the above are answered in the positive.

One excellent way to tag gurney-bound patient at risk of falling is to create a fall risk sign and hang it from the IV pole.

Do not use the *Scale* for infants or children.

Jan

THE INTERDISCIPLINARY CONSULTATION TEAM

All patients who initially score at high risk of falling should be reviewed, case by case by an interdisciplinary team. The purpose of such a review should be: (1) to reduce the patient's falls score (and therefore reduce the risk of the patient falling); (2) to prevent a fall by identifying appropriate fall prevention strategies; and (3) to prevent reoccurrence if the patient has fallen in the past. As mentioned in Chapter 1, the team should consist of the fall prevention clinical nurse specialist (as chairperson), the patient's primary nurse, a geriatrician, a physical therapist, a pharmacist, and an occupational therapist. Ad hoc members may include the patient (if oriented) or the patient's next-of-kin, and the patient's physician.

Dear Jan,

Most of our patients score high risk of falling on the *MFS*. Should we increase the cut-off score?

Sally

———

Hi Sally,

If most of your patients score at risk, that means they are at risk of falling. Often these patients are clustered in one area, such as in a stroke unit or a psychogeriatric unit. The scale is correct; they are all at risk of falling. Do not increase the cut-off score, but do provide protections and prevention strategies for all of those at risk.

Jan

PEDIATRIC FALLS

What about children? The problem is that falling is not a possibility for an infant who cannot walk. If you have a baby in your fall data set, it MUST, by definition, be an error! The baby must have been dropped, and a drop is not a fall. Next, falling is a natural developmental activity in toddlers. Toddlers experience standing falls all the time, usually without consequences. It would be absurd to try and score them with the fall risk assessment. Now toddlers do experience serious injuries when they climb and fall from heights, such as from windows or balconies, but these are a different type of fall, with different types of interventions needed, and they are outside the scope of this study. Children may fall when experiencing a seizure—an unanticipated physiological fall—again something that cannot be predicted with a fall risk scale.

Remember we are interested in *anticipated* physiological falls— falls that can be predicted and for which interventions may be used. Children do have anticipated physiological falls, but they do not experience injury until they are old enough and heavy enough to have an impact that will cause injury. The *MFS* was not developed with children in the sample (we started sampling at 18 years of age), so I have no reason to expect that it will "work" with children, although some investigators try (see Razmus, Wilson, Smith, & Newman, 2006).

However, as the Joint Commission has stated that for accreditation all patients must be scored, there are some risk assessment tools that were developed especially for children. I list them here, but have not used them in trials and have no information on their performance.

1   Falls Assessment Form—Children's Hospital Central California (Cooper & Nolt, 2007)
2   Graf, E. (2004). General risk assessment for pediatric in-patient falls scale (GRAF_PIF). Fall risk assessment tool, Children's Memorial Medical Center. Federal Copyright received 2005.
3   *Humpty Dumpty Scale.* Miami Children's Hospital.
4   *Little Schmidy Fall Score* (Adapted from the Schmid Fall Score tool for UCSF Children's Hospital) (2005) UCSF Medical Center.

REFERENCES

Cooper, C. L., & Nolt, J. D. (2007). Development of an evidenced-based pediatric fall prevention program. *Journal of Nursing Care Quality, 22* (2), 107–112.

McCollam, M. E. (1995). Evaluation and implementation of a research-based falls assessment innovation. *Nursing Clinics of North America 30*(3), 507–514.

Morse, J. M., Morse, R. M., & Tylko, S. J. (1989). Development of a scale to identify the fall-prone patient. *Canadian Journal on Aging, 8*(4), 366–377.

Razmus, I., Wilson, D., Smith, R., & Newman, E. (2006). Falls in hospitalized children. *Pediatric Nursing, 32*(6), 568–572.

5 Intervention: Fall Prevention and Protection

Chapter 2 described how to make the environment safer to help prevent accidental falls. In this chapter, we will first discuss strategies provided to all patients, regardless of their fall scores. These *routine fall intervention strategies* are simply standard nursing measures provided to all patients to increase their general comfort, but which also happen to reduce fall risk. Second, we will discuss the protective strategies provided to patients who have experienced unanticipated physiological falls. Finally, we will discuss the preventive and protective intervention strategies for patients who score at risk of anticipated physiological falls. Because there is some variance of risk according to patient typology, some of these strategies are particular to some patient care areas.

ROUTINE FALL INTERVENTION STRATEGIES

These routine fall interventions strategies are provided to all patients who are admitted to the hospital, but they warrant listing as fall intervention strategies because even if all patients cannot use all of these

71

strategies (because some strategies depend on the patient state and condition), they are considered basic nursing procedures.

Orientation

All patients admitted to a unit receive an orientation to the unit, along with instructions as to their freedom to move about. For instance, if they are on bed rest, they are informed that they must stay in bed and told whether they have bathroom privileges or must call the nurse for assistance if they need to go to the toilet. They are shown where the bathroom is and, if a shower is not provided in their room, they are shown where that is. They are instructed about use of the bathroom— for instance, if they may shower unassisted or must notify a nurse for assistance; where the toilet is, and if they may get up for the bathroom alone or call for assistance. They are taught about meal hours and, if on a special diet or fluid intake, what they may or may not eat or drink. They are given a tour or told about the layout of the unit, including where to find the patient lounge. They are given an overview of the daily routine, when meals are served, and when the doctors' rounds occur.

Call Bells

Nurses are required to demonstrate how to call for the nurse, and when to use the call bell. If the patient is bed-bound, nurses are required to keep the bell close to the patient at all times. Make certain the patient is able to push the button to call the nurse—if the patient has had a stroke, is disabled, or has a hand injury, request a call bell that may be activated some other way, such as an air activated one that works by blowing on it. If the patient is cognitively impaired, he or she will not remember to use the bell, and so their bed *must* have a bed alarm, and it must be placed in the unit where nurses can monitor the patient; the patient must be checked at least hourly.

While discussing call bells, do not forget to include instruction about the emergency call bells in the bathrooms. Tell patients that if they call (shout) out, they probably will not be heard—they must press the buzzer/bell/button, and they must not hesitate to do so if they feel in the least bit dizzy. "Call before you fall," should be the motto—not to "use the call bell on the way to the floor."

Footwear

All patients must have safe footwear, regardless of gait and ability to move about. The admitting nurse must check that the patient has slippers that fit his or her feet well, are easy to put on and to remove, yet are not of the "scuff" type that flop about the heel. They must have nonskid soles. The hem of the patient's pajamas, nightgown, or robe must not drag on the ground and interfere with walking.

Bed

When the patient's bed is in the down position, the patient should be able to sit on the bed and have the balls of his or her feet on the floor. It is not necessary for the entire foot to be flat on the floor, but the patient must be able to safely reach to the floor to get out of bed safely. If the patient cannot do this, order a low bed. Do not use a step stool, for this provides another hazard and tends to tip. Even if the patient is on bed rest, order a low bed. Ordering bed rest is no guarantee that the patient will not attempt to get out of bed—or may have permission to do so at some point—and the bed MUST be at a safe height. The patient should never have to jump to reach the floor.

Bathrooms

If the patient has trouble rising from the toilet, provide a raised seat. Patients who need a raised toilet seat have various problems: tall patients with an abdominal wound; patients who have had knee or hip surgery or who have joint stiffness such as arthritis or Parkinson's disease; patients who must not exert themselves, such as those with cardiac problems; and even patients with problems with their arms or hands who cannot pull on the rails to lift themselves from the toilet. Some patients may need a bedside commode, or a urinal, particularly at night. Tell the patient how often the night nurse will be coming into his or her room on night rounds. Ask what times he or she gets up to use the bathroom at night, and if they want to be awakened and assisted to the toilet.

Night Lighting

Show patients the location of the light switches and where the night-lights are located, so they may move about at night with minimal uncertainty. Make certain that at night they have everything they need within reach.

Patient's Walking Aids

Often patients come into the hospital with their own cane, crutches, walkers, or wheelchairs. Inspect these to make certain they are safe and, if you consider them to be substandard, replace them with hospital supply. A patient must not be allowed to use his or her own cane if the tip is defective and worn; likewise for a wheelchair with inadequate brakes or footrests that will not stay up when the patient stands.

Family Involvement in Care

With patient's permission, the family should be aware of the unit layout, the patient's routine, and any restrictions (especially on diet, fluid intake, and mobility). If the patient is a child or if the patient is cognitively impaired, this family link is very important. Some hospitals use family members as "sitters," that is, use family members to watch that the patient does not get out of the bed or chair and to call the nurse if she or he becomes restless and needs the toilet. If your hospital permits such sharing of responsibility, there must be some type of orientation for family members. This should include at least a brochure outlining their responsibilities, so that they do not, for instance, go to the cafeteria and leave the patient unattended without letting the nurse know of their departure.

Foreign Language

If the patient does not speak English and cannot comprehend instructions, a translator must be provided. Explain to the translator that you will need to know if the patient has understood his or her instructions about the bathroom and how the patient assesses his or her abilities. For this reason, it is important that the translator translate the *MFS* questions to the patient—and their responses—directly.

Summary

Clearly, in addition to the strategies outlined in the chapter on accidental falls (Chapter 2), there are basic routine fall interventions that must be available to all patients. These need to be adapted according to each patient's needs and abilities. These ensure basic interventions from falling for all patients.

UNANTICIPATED PHYSIOLOGICAL FALLS

Although theoretically we do not know if a patient will have an unanticipated physiological fall until they fall for the first time, often we may suspect that a patient may fall and can take precautions against that event. For instance, a patient may be considered seizure-prone and be placed on seizure medications. In such an instance, it would be appropriate to expect a fall to occur during a seizure and to give the patient a helmet to prevent head injury should this occur. If an elderly patient complains of her knee "giving way," give her a cane or a walker—something to support her should it indeed give way, thereby avoiding a fall and possible fractured hip. Suggest to the patient that she install a grab bar in her shower and beside her toilet at home, so she has something to hold on to and can support herself if needed. Stabilize furniture that may be used to hold on to, if necessary.

Patients often suddenly faint or have a hypotensive episode, perhaps as a result of getting up from the bed too quickly or from a drug reaction. Again, while the first episode cannot be predicted, the patient must be warned that if he feels dizzy to immediately call for help, and sit or lie down. If the patient is frail and has fallen heavily, give the patient hip protectors to wear to prevent injury should a second fall occur. If you suspect that the fall was related to the medications that the patient was receiving, notify the physician and request a pharmacy consultation.

In summary, while some unanticipated physiological falls may be suspected and prepared for, others may be a matter of protecting the patient from injury should a second fall occur. Protection from injury with recurrence is most important. For many falls, the identification of the cause and consultation with the physician and pharmacist is also crucial for the prevention of a second fall.

PHYSIOLOGICAL ANTICIPATED FALLS

Your patient has scored *at risk of falling.* Now what?

Knowing how to intervene for the fall-prone patient is one of the most difficult clinical problems in nursing.[1] The conundrum is that it is very difficult to ensure patient safety without causing harm in other ways. For instance, if the patient is restrained to prevent him or her from climbing out of bed and falling, these restraints themselves may cause harm—immobility has its own physical consequences and re-straints violate patients' rights and are considered unethical. The most serious consequence from using restraints is that the patient may be-come tangled in the restraints and die from asphyxiation. Therefore, restraint use as a prevention from falling should only be a last resort and used only with a physician's order. Some institutions use "sit-ters"—that is, staff who are hired specifically to sit beside the bed to watch the patient to ensure they do not try to get out of bed and fall. Sitters, as a solution to preventing a fall do solve the problem in that patients should not fall while being observed, but the use of sitters may be very expensive. (It is not uncommon in the United States for medical centers to budget more than $1,000,000/year for sitters). Us-ing a family member as a "sitter" is not a practical solution, as family members are often unwilling, are untrained, and often unreliable. Therefore, they cannot be responsible for fall prevention. They may not realize the risk of harm from a fall and may "step out" for a mo-

---

[1] I thank Mary Watson, Pat Quigley, and Charlotte Pooler for their assistance and insights regarding fall intervention strategies.

ment. Of greatest concern, hospitals are not constructed for the provision of safe care. For instance, most acute care hospitals do not have an enclosed area for patients to safely wander, making the nursing surveillance of the elderly wandering patient almost impossible.

Fall prevention programs, such as exercises, balance training programs, and tai chi are slow to become effective (for instance, it takes at least 3 months for a patient's gait to improve) and are, therefore, of limited value in the acute care setting, where the length of stay is frequently 3 days or less.

> Fall protection strategies protect the patient from injury should a fall occur.

The other approach to falls is to reduce the risk of injury should a patient fall. Fall *protection* became increasingly important with the *Release Restraints* movement—the organization that had, as its goal, freedom for the elderly.

Fall protective devices include equipment such as bed alarms that lessen the risk of falls by alerting the staff when a patient attempts to get out of bed or hip pads that provide padding should a patient fall, reducing the risk of a hip fracture, but both are unreliable and prone to "malfunction" because of human failure. The patient may move too quickly for a nurse to catch the patient, the patient may have removed the hip pad, the staff may not be able to respond

> Because residents fall in a variety of situations and these falls are due to innumerable causes, there cannot be one routine care plan to prevent falls. Fall intervention must be individually prescribed.

to the alarm in time to prevent the fall or, for some reason, may not have put the hip pad on the patient. Despite these frustrations, fall intervention—protection and prevention—cannot be omitted. To rate patients at risk of falling and not have any plan for fall intervention is a serious mistake. Also, providing only one intervention method, such as placing the onus on the nurse to "watch the patient," is totally inadequate.

> Most of the falls occur while the patient is getting out of bed. Beds must be kept in the low position except when care is being administered to the patient.

Further, because residents fall in a variety of situations and these falls are due to innumerable causes, there cannot be one routine care plan to prevent falls. Fall interventions must be individually prescribed.

The next section discusses fall interventions as *prevention strategies* and *protection strategies.*

> Fall interventions strategies are preventive or protective.

Whenever fall risk or fall interventions differ by care areas, this will also be discussed. Strategies are sorted by the categories as they are scored on the *Morse Fall Scale* (*MFS*).

However, while the *Scale* itself cannot be used prescriptively, the broad categories of scoring provide clues about how one should proceed for prevention. An overview is provided in Table 5.1.

Table 5.1

FALL INTERVENTION STRATEGIES BY *MFS* ITEM

MORSE FALL SCALE ITEM	ASSESSMENT GOAL	INTERVENTION STRATEGY	
		PREVENTIVE STRATEGY	PROTECTIVE STRATEGY
1. History of falling	To prevent recurrence of fall	Expect a 2nd fall; develop a strategy to prevent recurrence—at the same time with the patient doing the same activity. Develop patient-specific fall-intervention plan	Alert staff about the circumstances of the 1st fall. Conduct 2 hourly rounds.
2. Secondary Diagnosis	To determine interactions from polypharmacy	Consult with physician and pharmacy. Adjust medications accordingly.	
3. Gait	To assess impairment of gait and balance	Refer to PT for exercise program or tai chi. Walk regularly. Provide low bed. Safe route to bathroom—handholds? Rail? Stable furniture?	*Weak gait:* Remind to use call bell for assistance when getting out of bed; Use handrail Plan route

FALL INTERVENTION STRATEGIES BY *MFS* ITEM (*continued*)

MORSE FALL SCALE ITEM	ASSESSMENT GOAL	INTERVENTION STRATEGY	
		PREVENTIVE STRATEGY	PROTECTIVE STRATEGY
		Inform family about limitations and plan for fall intervention	*Impaired gait:* Gait belt when walking Provide assistance Use hip protectors Top side rail up to assist with mobility If noncompliant, use bed alarm
4. Ambulatory aid	To assess appropriate aids;	Avoid "rushing to bathroom"—check bowel and bladder function. Needs a walking aid? Provide appropriate aids (this will reduce the fall score). Aids used correctly? In reach?— Teach.	If wheelchair user, observe transferring technique
5. IV	To maximize safe ambulation; reduce urinary urgency	Assess for fluid balance, hypotension If using pole as walking aid, provide walker If urinary urgency, wake at 2 am for toileting	Remind about physical limitations
6. Mental status	Improve orientation and acceptance of changed abilities	Frequent observations, place bed in room near nursing station Two hourly "comfort" rounds Implement bowel and bladder program Involve family for observations, planning care	Frequent reorientation and reminders Door alarm Do not leave unattended in diagnostic areas *If gait also impaired,* Use bed alarm, chair alarm and hip protectors Use sitter Indicate fall risk on sign

INTERVENTIONS AS PREVENTION STRATEGIES AND PROTECTION STRATEGIES

History of Falling

Fall Interventions for Patients Who Have Had a Previous Fall

On admission, if the patient or relatives tell you that there was a previous fall within the past 3 months, try to elicit details about the type of fall, the time of day, and what the patient was doing when he or she fell. From this information, we are trying to identify the type of fall, because if the fall was an anticipated physiological fall (and the patient still scores at risk of falling), it is very likely that the patient will fall again *doing the same thing* at *about the same time of day.* If nurses have this information, they can take measures to prevent reoccurrence.

If, for instance, the relatives tell you that grandfather gets out of bed every night at 3 AM, then the night nurse can wake and assist him to the toilet at 2 AM, thereby preventing a recurrence of a fall.

> In 55% of cases, the first and second falls occurred in similar circumstances, often at the same time of day.

What was the patient doing when he or she fell? We are interested in fall–prone behavior—trying to identify patients who take risks, who do not follow instructions, and, for instance, try to get to the bathroom by themselves. Fall-prone behavior, behavior that puts the patient at risk of a fall or injury, is sometimes easy to identify and to correct.

If the previous fall was caused by a seizure, then protective strategies can be made, such as a helmet to prevent head injury upon a reoccurrence.

Repeated Falls: Has the Patient Fallen Before?

Of course, if the patient falls in the hospital, the fall score changes with this item checked. Record the time and circumstances of the fall, so the nurses who will subsequently care for this patient will be able to take steps to prevent recurrence.

Secondary Diagnosis: Fall Interventions

Recall that this item on the *MFS* is an index for medications, or polypharmacy. If polypharmacy is a fall risk, often the patient will also score on gait (weak or impaired) and on mental status. This is particularly problematic with patients in psychiatry, where their gait is often weak or impaired from their condition (e.g., the gait of depression), as well as their medication's action and interactions.

Intervention consists of consultation with the pharmacist and the physician. If drug interactions and reactions are introducing a fall risk, it is important that, if possible, the medications be adjusted.

Gait: Fall Interventions

Fall Interventions for Patients Who Score as Weak Gait

Ensure that the environment is safe and that handholds—wall rails—are available between the bed and the bathroom. Remind the patient to call (or ring) for assistance when getting out of bed. Provide assistance for the patient when walking if needed. These patients sometimes have a cane or a walker—especially if their gait is sometimes impaired. Ensure that they know how to use their walking aids correctly, that they park it close to their bed or chair when they rest, and that they do not carry their canes or walkers.

Fall Interventions for Patients Who Score Impaired Gait

These patients usually have both an impaired gait and balance and cannot walk without assistance. They usually have walking aids (see the next section). Therefore, in addition to the interventions for a weak gait, many other interventions must be provided to ensure their safety.

Gait belts for walking: When assisting these patients to walk, gait belts must always be used to ensure that the person assisting the patient has an adequate grip to support the *person.*

Hip protectors: Hip protectors are underwear that is padded, usually with firm foam, over both hips. These are made in many sizes (small to oversize) and in male and female sizes. The assumption is that if the patient falls, the pad over the hip will protect the person from a fractured hip. When initially introduced, these were considered most effective. However, as further studies were conducted, meta-analyses revealed less success in the prevention of fractured hips (Parker, Gillespie, & Gillespie, 2005).

Floor mats: Floor mats are pads made of firm rubber that are placed beside the bed. If the patient falls while climbing out of the bed, the mat provides some protection by cushioning the impact on the floor, therefore protecting the patient from a fractured hip. The edges of the mat are usually beveled, so that walkers and other equipment can move on to the mat and support the patient at the bedside.

While these mats do provide protection if the patient is climbing out of bed, they are less safe when the patient is climbing into bed. The "boggy" surface of the mat may catch on the patient's slippers and drag, further impeding the gait. The beveled edge may catch on walkers and cause the patient to stumble. As these mats are large and difficult to slide under the bed, they are only partly successful as an intervention—providing protection when patients are getting out of bed, but not getting in.

Supervision/nursing surveillance: These patients must be monitored and not left on the toilet where they may try to stand unassisted.

Bed/chair alarms: If the patient is restless, noncompliant, or confused and may exit the bed or chair unassisted, bed or chair alarms must be used (see *mental status*).

Assist with transferring: These patients will not be able to rise from the chair easily without assistance. Nurses should assist them to rise from a chair or get out of bed and move to the chair or bathroom.

Side rails: Side rails are important in that they help the patient turn over in bed, provide a handhold to help the patient sit up in bed, and stabilize the patient as s/he sits on the edge of the bed and stands. They therefore assist the patient with mobility. However, a side rail can also be a hazard. Side rails must never be used to "keep a patient in bed" for the patient will simply climb over the top of the rail (and, therefore, have further to fall and increased injury) or climb over the end of the bed (which is a vertical cliff). A safe route must always be left by leaving at least one of a split side rail down for the patient to leave the bed.

Walking Aid: Fall Interventions

If patients are prescribed a walking aid, it is imperative that they use it properly. Often canes are used not as a support for walking, but as an implement to reach a piece of paper or article that has fallen on the floor, or worse, to hit another resident. When attempting to sit, patients park their walkers, reach for their seats, and walk to sit down, rather than backing into their seat and using the walker to lower themselves into the chair. Walkers are not "parked" correctly, but left some distance from the chair, so that the patient must walk to the walker.

Of concern is the patient who is admitted with an impaired gait in the middle of the night or over the weekend because the staff does not have access to walking aids when physical therapy is closed. This is unacceptable, as the patient cannot ambulate without holding on to the furniture—which in hospitals is often placed too far apart to provide a safe route the to the bathroom.

> Walking aids must always be available to the staff.

If the staff find itself with such a patient, put a commode at the bedside and a bed alarm on the bed. It is imperative that you know when this patient is going to get out of bed. Also if the patient has an impaired mental status, use a bed/chair alarm to alert staff when the patient is getting out of bed, for these patients will not use walking aids correctly.

Fall Interventions

As noted in the discussion of the *Scale* development, we do not know exactly why this item was significant on the *Scale*. Initially, we suggested that the patients who had an IV were "sicker" than those without. Since that time, by examining patient falls with serious injury, we found that these patients who fell and were injured between 2 AM and 4 AM were not confused patients, but rather surgical patients. I believe the explanation is that these are surgical patients who are given an analgesic and something to help them sleep at bedtime. The IV continues to run. About 3 AM, these patients wake with a full bladder, need to micturate urgently, and because of the analgesic, feel well. They get out of bed, stand, and try to walk, but their reflexes do not work as well as they should and these patients fall hard. In these free falls, patients do not "break the fall" with their arms. These are falls that fracture bones—their arms (if they fall forward or sideways), their skull (if they fall backward), their ribs (if they hit something as they are falling). They are hard falls: they make a resounding crash in the unit, an unmistakable, dreadful sound.

The main intervention is to EXPECT that your patients will wake up with a full bladder about 3 AM. **Night nurses must wake postoperative patients at 3 AM and assist them to the bathroom (or give them a bedpan) and assist them back to bed.** If the patient is known to have frequency of micturition, then even every 1 or 2 hourly rounds, it may be necessary to assist the patient to the bathroom (Meade, Bursell, & Ketelsen, 2006). If these patients are unfamiliar with their environment, they may find that they cannot make it across the doors to get to the bathroom. Some form of night-light may be required to ensure that they walk in the right direction and do not fall over furniture or another object in the room.

Mental Status: Fall Interventions for Patient With Impaired Mental Status

These patients are typically elderly medical or surgical patients with sundowner's syndrome who cannot remember to "call" the nurse for assistance, but they may also be elderly patients who temporarily "forget where they are" in the night, younger patients who refuse to comply with the nurse's orders, or young men who are embarrassed to have a nurse waiting to assist them on the toilet and try to sneak out of bed without being caught. They may be patients with urinary urgency or diarrhea and, in their rush, forget to call the nurse for assistance.

Remember that several factors will assist with the fall intervention program. The first is communication among staff members, both verbally and in a report. Falling is sometimes the results of poor habits, and nurses, recognizing those patterns, must communicate them to other staff members. Similarly, communicating fall risk is important—not only high risk, but the patient's actual scores. This is done in some institutions by placing a sign, a falling star for instance, outside the patients door or, if the patient is a new admission, by hanging the sign on the IV pole, so that as the patient is transferred from emergency to x-ray on the gurney, the sign goes with the patient, alerting all. The assumption underlying the use of such signs is that fall interventions are the responsibility of all hospital employees. If, for example, a patient is getting out of bed unassisted and a staff member walking beside the door sees the patient, he or she is responsible for supporting and standing beside the patient until assistance arrives.

MONITORING INDIVIDUALS WHO FALL: IDENTIFYING PATTERNS

Repeated falls are not random events. Examination of the circumstances and time of repeated falls revealed that in 55% of the cases, the first and second fall occurred in similar circumstances (i.e., the patient was repeating the same activity), often at approximately the same time of day (Morse, Tylko, & Dixon, 1985). These patterns of falling become clear when examining data from a patient's chart:

Fall #1:	2:35 p.m.	Patient fell while climbing out of bed unassisted.
Fall #2:	3:10 a.m.	Patient found on floor beside bed. Disoriented.
Fall #3:	2:45 p.m.	Patient climbed out of bed unassisted. Slipped on urine.
Fall #4:	1:50 p.m.	Patient went to bathroom unassisted. Patient fell from commode.

From the above, it is clear that the nursing intervention should be to ensure that the patient empties his bladder prior to his nap and is awakened to be taken to the bathroom during nap time and again at 2 AM. Therefore, when a patient falls, it is important to make the staff aware of the fall, including the time and the circumstances of the fall, to prevent reoccurrence.

Fall Risk in Special Care Areas

Surgical Patients

Patients who are admitted for scheduled surgery are usually admitted with a normal gait. After a general anesthetic, all patients have a weak gait. If the surgery was major, their gait may be impaired. In the days following surgery, as the patient becomes stronger, the fall score should be reduced. It is imperative that these patients are scored at least twice daily.

Obstetrics

Following delivery, maternity patients often have a hypovolemic episode and faint on the floor. The first time out of bed or the first shower postdelivery are the periods most at risk. Advise patients that they may feel faint when they get up and should sit down if they feel dizzy. This risk is increased if the patient has been on bed rest for some time prior to delivery or has had a multiple birth.

Psychiatry

These patients are at risk of falling because of their response to their illness, as well as the effects of their medications. For instance, depression suppresses spontaneous movement, and the gait of a depressed person looks lumbering and awkward. A manic person might move too quickly, almost carelessly, and fall. These problems are increased by medications, which have side effects that further increase fall risk. They may cause tremors, spatial disorientation, dizziness, and so forth. A final challenge for the psych nurse is that many fall interventions introduce their own hazards—the bed alarm may have an electric cord—something that is considered a suicide risk in the psychiatric units. In addition, the nurses must decide if the patient had a real fall, or if they "fell" as an attention-getting strategy.

Medicine

Compared with surgical patients, the scores of medical patients are relatively stable, improving gradually over the course of the stay, and their condition improves.

Emergency Department

One of the difficult things to determine in the unit is to decide who to score when the unit is very busy. Regulations state that everyone is to be scored within 4 hours. I recommend that priority be given to those with an impaired gait (including the inebriated), and those with an impaired mental status. In this way, one would be triaging those most at risk and providing protective strategies in the most timely fashion.

Intensive Care

Score patients who get out of bed and patients who are restless. Do not bother scoring those patients who are not at risk of falling: those who are paralyzed and those who are unconscious.

Psychogeriatrics

These patients have the highest risk of falling. They have weak or impaired gaits and impaired mental status. They are often restless and need to ambulate, yet do not use their ambulatory aides correctly. There are bed alarms that may be programmed with a voice saying, "Get back into bed Mr. _____," rather than sounding an alarm. You can even record a relative's familiar voice on the machine, so as not to startle the patient. Use all your excellent nursing skills to settle these patients—make certain they have a comfortable chair, have been toileted, pain assessed, exercised, and back rubbed.

The most vulnerable patients and the most difficult to care for are those with end stage Alzheimer's. They often weigh less that 90 pounds, are incoherent, nonweight bearing, and pluck with their hands. Previously they were nursed on a Vail bed (i.e., one with cot-sides and even a roof) but these have been withdrawn.

Forensics

When patients who normally have a normal gait wear leg shackles, always score the gait as *weak*. Patients who are shackled cannot take a normal stride, and the weight of the chains and the short length impair the gait. When the patient is weak with illness or injury, the shackles may impede the gait enough as to rate it as impaired.

THE FALL

If a patient does fall, the fall may or may not result in an injury; if an injury occurs it may or may not be serious; if the injury is serious, it may or may not result in permanent disability or the death of the patient and litigation against the nurse, the physician, and the hospital administration. Falls are a serious problem that will become worse as the number of elderly increase, as the "baby boomer" generation matures.

We believe that falls are not a random event—they can be predicted. We also believe that whether or not a patient is injured when he or she falls is not a random event, but one that can be prevented.

When at patient falls, regardless of whether the patient is injured, a huge amount of activity should be set in motion. First, the nurse examines the patient for injury. Even if there is no apparent injury, s/he should notify the physician and the family. The nurse also notifies her supervisor and completes an *incident report form*. The fall is also charted on the patient's charts.

Using the Fall Reports

Many quality assurance departments file and tabulate the *incident report forms*, produce reports, and do little else. I would encourage them to do something else—to use the reports as a *diagnostic tool*.

When they receive the reports, the quality assurance personnel should, along with the fall clinical specialist nurse, go and look at the physical location where the fall occurred. They must inspect the area for unevenness in the flooring; inspect the lighting; and ask, was there a handhold? How did this happen? They must try to re-create the incident.

I can hear you asking, "But physiological anticipated falls are not accidents. Why are you looking for an environmental cause?"

You are right—but remember that physiological anticipated falls are an accident about to happen. Patients with an impaired gait cannot lift their feet very far off the floor at all and trip more easily than a person with a normal gait. We have the responsibility to protect our patients.

If any environmental cause at all can be found, it must be immediately remedied—not just in that particular room, but everywhere in the hospital where that problem is evident. When hospitals are being built, they replicate each room, over and over, so that if there is a problem in one room, it will be in them all.

Next, the quality assurance officer places a green dot recording the place of the fall on a hospital map—rather as tennis broadcasts on TV show the position of the ball for each serve. This will show fall "hot spots" very quickly, and help focus the inquiry.

Let me give you an example. One hospital had floor covering changes—the rooms were linoleum and the hallways carpeted. The flooring specialists had placed a wooden "bead" covering the join in the doorway. This was less than half an inch high, but it was enough to trip a person with an impaired gait. When I pointed out the problem, staff said that they had falls there previously, but it had not been noticed—and they said that they had even stubbed their toe on this wood.

Solving the puzzle of falls is rather like being a detective—use all the data you can, and use it well. Repairs do not come without costs, but these costs must be easier to manage than patient injury, the legal system, and one's conscience.

One final word—do these fall interventions work?

In a recent meta-analysis of eight fall intervention studies, Coussement, De Paepe, Schwendimann et al. (2008) concluded that there is no conclusive evidence that fall interventions programs can reduce patient falls, but that more studies are needed. Only two of the studies in this meta-analysis included data on injury rates, so that the focus also needs to move from fall rate reduction to injury rates. Therefore, since the jury is still out, we do the moral thing, the only thing to do—continue with fall intervention programs.

REFERENCES

Coussement, J., De Paepe, L., Schwendimann, R., Denhaerynck, K., Dejaeger, E., & Milisen, K. (2008). Interventions for preventing falls in acute- and chronic-care hospitals: A systematic review and meta-analysis. *Journal of the American Geriatric Society, 56,* 29–36.

Meade, C. M., Bursell, A. L., & Ketelsen, L. (2006). Effects of nursing rounds on patients call light use, satisfaction and safety. *American Journal of Nursing, 106* (9), 58–70.

Parker, M. J., Gillespie, W. J., & Gillespie, L. D. (2005). Hip protectors for preventing hip fractures in older people. *Cochrane Database of Systematic Reviews 2005* Issue 3. Art No.: CD001255. DOI 10.1002/14651858.CD001255pub3.

6   Conducting a Fall Assessment

A fall assessment should be conducted on all patients who score at risk of falling and repeated after a fall occurs to revise the fall risk score. Each of the three types of falls can be caused by a myriad of factors. Therefore, there are numerous strategies to prevent the fall. Identifying the cause of the fall requires observational and assessment skills on the part of the nurse and a consultation by a *multidisciplinary team* to identify possible physiological causes. It also requires regular checking of the environment for hazards that may have contributed to the fall. Finally, it requires developing a plan for the prevention of a subsequent fall.

COMPONENTS OF A FALL ASSESSMENT

Assessing the Patient's Physical Ability

This concerns the patient's ability to ambulate, rise, and get into a chair, to transfer between the bed and the chair, and to climb in and out of bed. It should also include an assessment of the patient's ability to toilet on his or her own—to sit on and rise from the commode, as well as to clean one's self, while managing night gowns, robes, and pajama pants, perhaps while holding onto the support rail.

Assessing the Patient's Mental Status

Assess the patient's assessment of his or her own abilities. Is s/he able to use the call bell? Is s/he willing to ask for assistance to get up of bed, and does s/he remember to do so? Is the patient aware that s/he is unable to move about the room without support or a walking aid? Does s/he remember to use the walking aid as instructed?

Assessing the Patient's Ability and Mode of Ambulation

In the hospital, we observed that the elderly often overestimated their own abilities. In their own homes, for instance, the elderly could move about by holding onto furniture and cross doorways by reaching for the far side of the door frame. But in the hospital, this unexpectedly becomes dangerous. In hospital, the doorways are built to accommodate gurneys and are, therefore, wider than those in the home. There are greater distances between pieces of furniture and, when the furniture is used as a support, it is often on wheels and slides away from the person who is using it as a support.

Therefore, observe how the person moves about the room. Does s/he reach for the support of furniture and "dive" across doorways reaching for the far door frame? If so, these patients must be given a walking frame to use for support and must be instructed in its use. Again, check to see if they use it consistently according to directions.

> Hospitals appear disproportionately large to the sick person.

Assessing the Patient's Ability to Sit

Check where the patient prefers to sit. Is the chair low and, therefore, difficult to rise from? On the other hand, if the patient has an impaired gait and is confused, staff may want the patient to sit in a chair that is difficult to get out of so the patient may be easier to monitor. Is the chair comfortable? Does the chair have arms that provide adequate leverage when the patient tries to rise? Watch the patient rise. Is the patient able to rise directly or does it take many "bounces," pushing on the arms of the chair, before the patient is upright? Is the chair stable or secure, or does it slide backward when the patient stands? When the patient stands, is s/he steady or does s/he need to immediately reach for support, even while continuing to reach back to the chair's armrest? Does the patient grab the support and clutch onto it, or does the patient simply rest his or her fingers on that support? Also, when they walk, observe their gait.

Assessing Wheelchair Use

When transferring, rising from, or sitting down, those who use wheelchairs are at most risk of falling.

Observe the patient transferring from the wheelchair to the bed, and vice versa. Does the patient bring the wheelchair as close as possible to the bed? Is there a height difference between the bed and the chair, and does the patient adjust the bed accordingly? Does the patient apply the brakes on the wheelchair? Is the bed braked? If the patient is weight bearing, are the leg rests and foot pedals moved out of the way so the patient can stand? Does the patient use a transfer board, and is it secure? If the patient has casts on his or her legs, is the wheelchair weighted to prevent tipping? Finally, is the wheelchair a comfortable fit considering the patient's size?

> When transferring, patients are at risk of falling.

Assessing Patient's Daily Routine

Understanding the patient's routine will provide insights into the times that the patient needs assistance to go to the bathroom or when the patient may be tired, weakest, and his/her gait most impaired. It provides important information about when the patient is awake and restless at night and for which periods during the day the patient may be most at risk and need to be toileted or exercised. On the other hand, it provides information about the patient's patterns and times of sleep when the nurses may be less vigilant.

Assessing Patient's Need for Exercise

Patients need to be exercised, and this routine is important to prevent muscle wasting and to prevent increasing weakness. Even if the patient needs the assistance of two nurses, it is recommended that patients are regularly walked to the toilet and back to their chair rather than using a wheelchair. Establishing this routine ensures that patients are exercised as well as toileted.

Assessing Things That "Settle" the Patient

Observe the patient to ascertain what the patient responds to. What calms or settles the patient? Ask the family what type of music the patient enjoys. Ensure that patients are warm enough because when patients are cold, they become restless.

When a Fall Occurs

When a fall occurs, first ensure the patient's condition. Assess the patient for injury, take vital signs, and, if necessary, apply first aid. If the patient is on anticoagulants and informs the physician and the charge nurse, begin postfall head injury checks as directed.

Complete the paperwork: When a fall occurs, the circumstances and events surrounding the fall should be recorded. Obtain as much information as possible from the patient and from witnesses about the cause of the fall. Record:

1   The circumstances surrounding the fall:
    - Where did the fall occur? Were there any environmental factors that may have contributed to the fall? Was it an accidental fall? Could a second fall be prevented by making modifications to the setting?

- What was the patient doing at the time of the fall? Was the patient getting out of or into bed? As soon as possible, have

  > Always identify the type of fall that occurred.

  the patient repeat the activity, while observing closely. If the patient's fall occurred while getting out of a chair, have the patient rise from the same chair. Observe if the chair was stable when the patient stood, where the patient parked his/her walker, and if the chair-walker transfer was correctly done. If the patient had to reach for the walker, consider if the patient was steady on rising and upright before beginning to walk, and so forth.
- Was there a "warning?" Did the patient feel that s/he was going to fall, or did the patient not realize what had happened until found on the floor?
- How did the patient fall? (i.e., did the patient try to break the fall, grab onto something to break the fall, or was it a "free fall" without even the patient's arms breaking the impact?).

2 Determine the type of fall, according to the classification of types of falls (Chapter 1). Was it an accidental, unanticipated physiological, or an anticipated physiological fall?

- If an *accidental fall*, identify the environmental factors that may have contributed to the fall.
- If an *unanticipated physiological fall*, examine the time, the circumstances, and possible physical conditions contributing to the fall.
- If it was an *anticipated physiological fall*, examine the patient's fall score and collect information on the pattern of the fall score to determine if there is a time when the patient is more likely to be at risk of falling.

3 Meet with appropriate members of the multidisciplinary team and identify remedial fall prevention strategies to prevent the fall from reoccurring.

- If it was an accidental fall, meet with the appropriate members of the multidisciplinary team. For instance, if the fall was due to a defective wheelchair, discuss with maintenance how the system of safety checks can be improved so that all wheelchairs are included in the schedule. Develop a plan to prevent recurrence.

■ If it was an unanticipated physiological fall, meet with the multidisciplinary team to determine how the patient's fall score may be reduced and to identify strategies to prevent reoccurrence. For example, if the patient was confused and was trying to get to the bathroom unassisted, review the patient's medications with the physician and the pharmacist for possible drug interactions that may contribute to the confusion. This intervention, if successful, would reduce the patient's fall score. Would preventive nursing measures, such as withholding bedtime fluids reduce the need to void at night? Or would regular toileting 1 hour prior to the time of the fall reduce the risk of reoccurrence? Would a bed alarm alert the staff in time to assist the patient? These preventative strategies would then be developed into a fall prevention plan, individualized according to the needs of that particular patient.

■ If it was an anticipated physiological fall, again meet with interdisciplinary team to see if the possible cause of the fall may be rectified. For instance, if the fall was caused by fainting, examine the patient to identify the probable cause of the fainting and develop a plan to prevent reoccurrence.

Finally, record the details of the fall and develop a care plan by identifying fall prevention strategies to prevent recurrence.

Evaluating the Effectiveness of the Program

HOW DO YOU KNOW IF YOUR FALL PROGRAM IS WORKING?

The most obvious way to evaluate your program is to track the number of falls monthly and the number of patient injuries. Unfortunately this is not as clear-cut as it sounds. The problems are complex.

First, whenever one starts a fall intervention program, everyone is enthusiastic about the program. In fact, just saying "go" may have the same effect on injury rates as an expensive intervention. This is the *Hawthorne effect*, and it is the bane of clinical research. However, if our change is real and extends from your interventions, over time, as you chart your statistics each month, the number of injuries should continue to decline or, at least, remain steady.

> Always focus on the number of injuries rather than on the number of falls.

The second problem, tracking the number of falls/1000 patient bed days, is more complex. At first you may be surprised (and not so pleased) to see the number of falls increase dramatically for the first few months, rather than decrease as you expected. This is a reporting error.

Before you commenced your program, reporting a fall was probably a haphazard activity at best. Reporting was probably considered an onerous task, associated with feelings of guilt and worry that it might reflect negatively on the nurse's record. Besides, the nurse may not actually be certain that the patient did fall—so she decides that it would be better if she did not report it. Thus, there is a lot of error in the fall database. But after the program has started and nurses realize that to have a patient fall is not something that may result in punishment but rather is an interesting event, all falls are suddenly reported, and the rate goes up. If your database has been "cleaned" and the nonfalls removed—and staff and visitor falls removed—the new rate will look even higher.

> The initial increase in falls may be due to a reporting error.

Remember it is just an artifact of starting a new program; the rate will eventually settled down. Draw a graph so that you can show the declining fall rate—such feedback provides the necessary encouragement for the staff.

But we are not out of the woods yet. The status quo for fall reporting can return very quickly. The fall clinical nurse researcher must constantly hold workshops, report the fall rates back to each unit, and keep fall consciousness at the forefront.

HOW DO YOU KNOW IF THE *MORSE FALL SCALE* (*MFS*) IS WORKING IN YOUR SETTING?

Is the patient population similar to the patients in the original study developing the *Scale*? Is the *MFS* working for you? Should the scale be validated in your setting?

These are difficult questions—and, by and large, I do not think it is necessary to reassess the *Scale* in each new setting. This is a standard required for psychological scales, and the *MFS* is not a psychological scale. Did your institution test the Glasgow coma scale and the APGAR scale prior to adopting these?

Furthermore, such an evaluation is difficult to do, for as soon as you rank someone as at risk of falling, then you are obligated to implement strategies to prevent the fall, and therefore prevent the dependent variable. Thus the evaluation is not valid and would show a low specificity with a large number of false positive ratings (i.e., patients rated as fall-prone, who did not fall).

There are many studies in the literature that have used this faulty design as well making other errors, hence invalidating the trial. Most commonly, these authors have used chart data in their trials, rather than examining the patient directly. I am stunned to see this problem constantly recurring, for I do not know how they are able to score *gait* and *mental status* from chart data. **The *MFS* cannot be scored from chart data, and any study that has evaluated the *MFS* using chart data is invalid.**

DOES THE *MFS* HAVE NORMS?

A prevalence study was conducted by Quigely et al. in 2006. All patients in the VA system in Florida and Puerto Rico (i.e., six medical centers) were scored using the *MFS* over a 2-day period (n=1819 patients). The researchers report the distribution of these scores by age, showing the rapid increase in scores over the age of 80; and they reported that the mean score for surgical patients was 47.3 (sd 25.64), and long term care 50.75 (sd 22.53). One could compare *MFS* mean scores in your institution with these reported scores.

In a second study, Schwendimann, De Geest, Milisen et al. (2006) administered the *MFS* to a large sample to determine the most appropriate cut off (or high risk) score. They explored every score in increments of 5 from 20 to 70, and concluded that a score of 55 had the most optimal sensitivity and specificity.

Therefore, do not set the high risk score over 55.

Sometimes, researchers who have used the *MFS* make recommendations for practice. For instance, occasionally, you find fall rates reported on the Internet. This is important for it means that the stigma for reporting fall rates is declining. However, when looking to compare your rates, make certain that the hospital is reporting using the same statistics (i.e., the same formula for fall and injury rate) and that your hospital populations are comparable. You may also look in the literature for reports of fall programs used in other hospitals (See Table 7.1).

Table 7.1 illustrates the difficulty in finding comparable rates. The alternative is to find a database offering benchmarking.

BENCHMARKING

For fall interventions, *benchmarking* is comparing your institutional fall rate and injury rate with other hospitals of a similar type.

The purpose of having such open standards is to enable comparison of fall rates in many ways: geographically, by patient type, and so forth, so that change (i.e., the lowering of fall rates) will occur more rapidly.

Table 7.1

FALL AND INJURY RATES FOR DIFFERENT PATIENT POPULATIONS

AUTHOR (DATE)	SETTING	FALL RATE (# FALLS/# PATIENT BED DAYS) × 1,000	INJURY RATE	COMMENTS
Barnett (2002)	General hospital	9.6	22%	England
Healey, et al. (2004)	Geriatric	17.99	4.42/1000 pt bed days	England
Hitcho, et al. (2004)	Medical Neurology	6.12 6.12	8%	USA
Schwendiman (2008)	Geriatrics Internal medicine Surgery	10.7 9.6 3.2	30.1% minor 5.1% major	Switzerland
von Rentein-Kruse, et al. (2007)	General	10.0	26.9%	Germany

In the United States, the largest database is the American Nurses Credentialing Center (ANCC) National Database on Nursing Quality Indicators sponsored by the American Nurses Association, and is situated at the University of Kansas, School of Nursing. In the creation of this database, the ANA had two goals:

> Benchmarking is a reasonable way to compare your rates with comparable hospitals.

- to provide comparative information to health care facilities for use in quality improvement activities
- to develop national data on the relationship between nurse staffing and patient outcomes

From the database, nurse executives may obtain such information as national averages for facilities of their size, significance tests, percentile ranking, and other statistical information to help them assess staffing and patient outcomes. (Visit: www.NursingWorld.org). As of February 2006, 899 hospitals were participating in the program (Nevada RN Information, February 2006).

Another alterative, if your hospital is a part of a consortium or chain, is to compare fall and injury rates by participating hospitals. Ideally, to make the statistics comparable, comparisons along some specific dimensions should be made. For instance, comparisons may first be made by hospitals of a similar size and second by comparing patient populations within each hospital. An example of such collaboration is that of the acute care hospitals in Massachusetts Hospital Association (for example, see http://www.patientsfirstma.org/nqf/NQFhospitals.cfm). All of these hospitals published their fall and injury rates, comparing them with the mean score of the consortium's combined scores (MHA/MONE patients first nurse-sensitive measure report, 2007). Thus, comparisons may be by hospital size (less than 100 beds, 100–199, 200–299, and so forth), by hospital types (rehabilitation, long-term care, acute, etc.), by clinical areas (adult critical, care units, adult surgical, medical, medical-surgical, and of forth), or combinations of these variables. For instance, Spaulding Rehabilitation Hospital reports a fall rate of 6.47/1,000 patient bed days and a peer group average of 5.05/1,000 patient bed days for the period from October 2006 to March 2007. At the same time, patient falls with injury were 1.46, and the peer group average was 0.84/1,000 patient bed days.

One final caution when benchmarking concerns comparing one's statistics with a group average. The results do not provide you with any definitive information: They do not tell you *why* your fall rate may be greater (or less) than that of other hospitals. The literature provides some clues, such as poor staffing levels or an older building, that are associated with hazards and falls, or even perhaps that your patients are *sicker*. The rationale for determining associations with the rates in a hospital should be determined by separate investigation.

Once the data are available, these data may be plotted on a graph, showing, for instance, your hospital's falls compared with at the national average and your target goal. Or the graph may display fall rates and injury rates each month for 1 year, displaying a trend that is decreasing as the fall rate drops.

REFERENCES

Barnett, K. (2002). Reducing patient falls in an acute general hospital. *The Foundation of Nursing Studies, 1*(1), 1–4.

Coussement, J., De Paepe, L., Schwendimann, R., Denhaerynck, K., Dejaeger, E., & Milisen, K. (2008). Interventions for preventing falls in acute- and chronic-care hospitals: A systematic review and meta-analysis. *Journal of the American Geriatrics Society. 56*(1), 29–36.

Healey, F., Monro, A., Cockram, A., Adams, V., & Heseltine, D. (2004). Using targeted risk factor reduction to prevent falls in older in-patients: a randomized controlled trial. *Age and Ageing, 33*, 390–395.

Hitcho, E., Krauss, M., Birge, S., Dunagan, W., Fischer, I., Johnson, S., et al. (2004). Characteristics and circumstances of falls in a hospital setting: A prospective analysis. *Journal of General Internal Medicine, 19*(7), 732–739.

MHA/MONE Patients First Nurse-Sensitive Measure Report (2007, October). *MHA/MONE Patients First Nurse-Sensitive Measure Report, Statistical Appendix.* Retrieved June 2, 2007, http://www.patientsfirstma.org/nqf/NQFhospitals.cfm.

Nevada RN Information. (2006, February). *NDNQI—National Database of Nursing Quality Indicators transferring data into quality care.* Retrieved April 10, 2008, from http://findarticles.com/articpaes/mi_qa4102/is_200602/ai_n1717021.

Quigley, P. A., Palacios, P., & Spehar, A. (2006). Veteran's fall risk profile. A prevalence study. *Clinical Interventions in Aging, 1*(2), 169–173.

Schwendimann, R., De Geest, & Milisen, K. (2006). Evaluation of the Morse Fall Scale in hospitalized patients. (Letter). Evaluation of the Morse Fall Scale in hospitalized patients. *Age & Ageing, 35*(3), 311–3.

Appendices

Researching
Patient Falls

Development of the
Morse Fall Scale

The procedure for developing the *Morse Fall Scale* (*MFS*) was briefly (1) establishing a database from 100 patients who fell and 100 randomly selected patients who had not fallen (*n*=200); (2) identifying the significant variables that differentiate those who fell from those who did not; (3) obtaining *Scale* weights for each item; (4) using the weights from these significant variables to calculate item values and to determine the *Scale* score that classifies patients at risk of falling; (5) computer testing the *Scale* on a simulated patient population (obtained from the original database); (6) estimating the reliability; and (7) establishing validity by randomly splitting the data set and repeating steps 2 to 4 on one half of the data, and, using discriminant analysis, testing the subsequently derived *Scale* variables on the other half of the data.

THE ESTABLISHMENT OF A DATABASE

The examination of 100 patients who fell and 100 controls (i.e., randomly selected patients who had not fallen) provided a database for the development of the *Scale*. A fall was defined as an event in which the patient came to rest on the floor (see Morris & Isaacs, 1980). This definition includes patients slipping from the chair to the floor, patients found lying on the floor and listed as fallen (i.e., falls in which a by-stander caught the patient and, although the impact of the fall was pre-vented, the patient was lowered on to the floor). Physiological and en-vironmental variables were collected from both groups and, for the fall group, information pertaining to the circumstances of the fall. Data were obtained from the patients' charts, by examining the patient, and by inspecting the environment. Comparisons were made using the chi-square test and the Kolmogorov-Smirnov two-sample test.

A comparison of patients who had fallen with the control group showed that the following variables were not significant: the gender of the patient, primary diagnosis, orthostatic hypotension, temper-ature, hemoglobin, presence of diarrhea or vomiting, method of void-ing, visual impairments, and hearing deficits. The control group was significantly younger than the fall group, and 58% of the patients that fell were between 65 and 89 years of age. It is of significance that those patients in the fall group were hospitalized longer ($p=0.02$), had fallen before ($p<0.0005$), had more than one diagnosis ($p<0.0005$), were confused ($p<0.0005$), had nocturia with urgency ($p=0.02$), had ab-normal skin turgor ($p=0.05$), had an IV ($p<0.0005$), used oxygen ($p=0.05$), and were less likely to experience pain that interfered with movement ($p=0.01$). The fall group were also more likely to have an abnormal gait ($p<0.0005$) and to require nursing assistance or crutches, a cane, or a walker when ambulating ($p<0.0005$) (Morse et al., 1987). A complete listing of variables included in this analysis is shown in Table A.1.

IDENTIFYING SIGNIFICANT VARIABLES

Discriminant analysis was used to classify individuals according to the criterion variable (i.e., whether or not the patient had fallen). The discriminant classification is based on an index derived from scores obtained from a set of discriminant variables. Six variables met the sig-nificant criterion of $F>.001$ as minimum tolerance level. These vari-

Table A.1

COMPARISON OF PATIENTS WHO FELL WITH RANDOMIZED CONTROLS: SIGNIFICANT AND NON-SIGNIFICANT VARIABLES

SIGNIFICANT VARIABLES	P	NON-SIGNIFICANT VARIABLES
Age	.000	Gender
Length of hospitalization	.002	
History of falling	.000	
Secondary diagnosis	.000	Primary Diagnosis
Mental status	.000	Height
Skin turgor	.002	Weight
Respirator: Use of O_2	.05	Diarrhea
Pulse rate	.02	Vomiting
Pain	.01	Bowel sounds
Nocturia with urgency	.05	Hemoglobin
IV therapy	.000	Orthostatic hypotension
Vision: use of lens	.04	
Gait	.000	
Walking aids	.000	
Side rails	.002	

ables included: history of falling (i.e., a previous fall); presence of a secondary diagnosis; use of intravenous therapy; type of gait (i.e., normal, weak, or impaired); the type and use of ambulatory aids; and mental status.

The variables were defined as follows:

History of Falling

This was coded as one if a previous fall was recorded during the present hospital admission or if there was an immediate history of physiological falls, such as from seizures or an impaired gait prior to admission.

Secondary Diagnosis

This was coded as one if more than one medical diagnosis was listed on the patient's chart. This variable was an index for polypharmacy.

We first searched for a drug that was correlated with falls and then a class of drugs, but neither was significant. What was correlated was polypharmacy and having more than one diagnosis is a rapid indice of that. Note that it does not matter what the second diagnosis is.

Ambulatory Aids

This was coded as zero if the patient walked without a walking aid (even if assisted by a nurse) or was on bed rest. If the patient used crutches, a cane, or a walker, this was coded as one; if the patient ambulated clutching onto the furniture for support, it was coded as two.

Intravenous Therapy

This was coded as one if the patient had an intravenous apparatus or a saline lock inserted.

Gait

The characteristics of the three types of gait were evident regardless of the type of physical disability. A normal gait is characterized by the patient walking with head erect, arms swinging freely at the sides, and striding unhesitatingly. It was coded as zero.

With a *weak gait* (coded as one), the patient is stooped but able to lift his or her head while walking. Support from furniture is sought, but this is a featherweight touch, almost for reassurance. The steps are short, and the patient may shuffle.

With an *impaired gait* (coded as two), the patient may have difficulty rising from the chair, attempting to rise by pushing on the arms of the chair and/or by "bouncing." The patient's head is down and, because the balance is poor, the patient grasps on to the furniture, a support person, or a walking aid, and cannot walk without this assistance. The steps are short, and the patient shuffles.

If the patient was in a wheelchair, the patient was scored according to the gait s/he used when transferring from the wheelchair to the bed.

Mental Status

In this study, mental status was measured by checking the patient's self-assessment of ambulatory ability. The patient was asked if s/he was able to go to the bathroom alone or if s/he needed assistance or if s/he was permitted to get up. If the patient's assessment was consistent with the ambulatory orders from the nursing staff, the patient was rated as normal and coded zero. If the patient's response was not consistent with these orders or if the patient's assessment was unrealistic, then the patient was considered to have *overestimated his/her own abilities,* to be *forgetful of limitations,* and was coded as one.

In this study, the dependent variable was dichotomous (i.e., each subject could be classified as either a faller or a control). Therefore, if a patient was randomly classified either in the fall group or in the control group, there would be a 50% probability of a correct classification.

When performing discriminant analysis, four groups are obtained, as follows (see Table A.2). In the study, the discriminant solution, using the six significant variables, correctly classified 78% of the fall group and 83% of the control group (total correct: 80.5%). This result is significantly greater than the 50% that would be expected to occur by chance. Results are shown in Table A.3. Standardized canonical correlation coefficients for each of the variables are shown in Table A.4. The Wilks' lambda (indicating the degrees of overlap between the two distributions) was .5829. An eigenvalue of .686 was obtained,

Table A.2

FOUR GROUPS OBTAINED BY DISCRIMINANT ANALYSIS

| PREDICTED GROUP | Actual Group | |
	FALL	CONTROL
Fall	Falls Correct (True Positive)	Controls Incorrect (False Positive)
Control	Falls Incorrect (False Negative)	Controls Correct (True Negative)

Table A.3

RESULTS OF DISCRIMINANT ANALYSIS

	Actual Group	
PREDICTED GROUP	FALL	CONTROL
Fall (*n*=100)	78 (39%)	17 (8.5%)
Control (*n*=100)	22 (11%)	83 (41.5%)

Table A.4

STANDARDIZED CANONICAL COEFFICIENTS

VARIABLE	COEFFICIENT
History of Falling	0.41111
Secondary Diagnosis	0.41949
Ambulatory Aid	0.49665
Intravenous Therapy	0.50162
Gait	0.34784
Mental Status	0.31223

indicating that 69% of the variance was accounted for between the two groups and the six variables accounted for 39.8% of the total variance (See Table A.4).

OBTAINING *SCALE* WEIGHTS FOR EACH ITEM

From the discriminant analysis output, the Fisher's linear function score was used to calculate the fall *Scale* weights for each item. The score was obtained for each discriminant variable for both the fall and the control groups. As shown in Table A.5, values obtained for the control group were subtracted from the values obtained for the fall group for each item. For the *Scale* to be optimally useful and scores easily

Table A.5

CALCULATION OF *SCALE* WEIGHTS

	Fisher's Linear Functions Score			
VARIABLE	FALL	CONTROL	FALL-CONTROL	*SCALE VALUE**
History of Falling	2.6004	0.0704	2.6708	25
Secondary Diagnosis	3.2857	1.7896	1.4961	15
Ambulatory Aid	1.7458	0.3662	1.3795	15
Intravenous Therapy	3.3969	1.1750	2.2219	20
Gait	1.3868	0.6230	0.7638	10
Mental Status	1.0360	-0.3477	1.3837	15

* Calculated as follows: Fall minus control multiplied by 10. Result was then rounded to nearest integer divisible by five.

calculated, these values were then multiplied by 10 and brought to the nearest integer divisible by five, provided this procedure did not interfere with the discriminant values of the test. This technique ensured greater reliability than the technique of improper linear modeling where *Scale* items are assigned equal values (Dawes, 1979) as, for example, is used in the Apgar scale (Apgar, 1953). These six items and values formed the *MFS*, with a maximum score of 125.

DETERMINING THE LEVEL OF RISK

The constant obtained from the Fisher's linear score (again, the constant score for the fall group minus the score for the control group) is the score used to determine risk of falling, separating high risk from low risk. Next, using the SPSSx frequencies program (augmented with "select if" and "compute" statements), the constant score was adjusted by single increments. The analysis was then repeated with each increment, and the percentages of cases correctly and incorrectly identified with each solution were obtained. Increasing the constant (the level of determining risk) has the effect of decreasing the false positives while increasing false negatives, or vice versa if the constant is decreased. As it was considered more important to reduce the number of false negatives (i.e., failing to identify a patient that was liable to fall) without greatly compromising the total percent correct, the final selection of the constant was a matter of judgment (Dawes, 1979; Lachenbruch, 1975).

COMPUTER TESTING OF THE *SCALE*

Next, using SPSSx facilities, the data set was weighted to resemble the hospital population according to the patients' risk of falling in the institution. As this institution had an average fall rate of 2.5 patient falls/1,000 patient bed days, the probability of a fall was 1:40 during an average 30-day stay. Thus, the database was increased to include 100 cases from the fall group and 4,000 controls. The discriminant analysis procedures were then repeated in the normalized data set.

The result of the discriminant analysis with the "normalized" population (i.e., 100 fallers and 4,000 controls) correctly classified 82.99% of the cases, as shown in Table A.6.

From the preceding data, the sensitivity of the *Scale,* or the rate of a correct decision is 78/100, or 78%. Thus, the positive predictive value is 78/(78+680)=10.3%. Conversely, the specificity of the *Scale,* or the rate of correct decisions for patients who have not fallen, is 3320/4000=83%, and the negative predictive value is 3320 (22+3320) = 99.2%.

Table A.6

RESULTS OF DISCRIMINANT ANALYSIS WITH "NORMALIZED" POPULATION

PREDICTED GROUP	Actual Group	
	FALL	CONTROL
Fall (*n*=100)	78 (1.9%)	680 (16.59%)
Control (*n*=100)	22 (0.54%)	3320 (80.98%)

ESTIMATION OF RELIABILITY

Interrater reliability was established with 21 nurses rating six patients. To ensure consistency, patients' gaits were videotaped, and this videotape was used for the scoring. Interrater reliability estimations for a five-item *Scale* was $r=.96$.[4] Scores for individual items were: history of falling and intravenous therapy, $r=1.0$; secondary diagnosis, $r=.99$; ambulatory aids, $r=.98$; and gait, $r=.82$.

A test for internal consistency revealed poor interitem correlations, with a coefficient alpha .16. This, combined with the results of analysis of variance ($f=71.34, p>.0001$), suggests that the items are relatively independent. However, as the *Scale* is only six items long, this is perhaps a necessary feature for measuring a multifaceted phenomenon.

ESTABLISHMENT OF VALIDITY

When developing the *Scale*, a major threat to validity was that the discriminatory power of the *Scale* was tested on the same population from which the *Scale* weights were obtained. This was remedied by randomly splitting the cases (using the nonnormalized data, $n=200$) and repeating the *Scale* construction procedures by obtaining *Scale* weights from 50% of the cases and retesting the discriminatory power of these weights on the remaining 50% of the cases.

Validation of the *Scale* by randomly splitting the data set did not alter the value of the weights obtained for the score variables. When tested on the remaining data ($n=102$, 54 fallers and 48 controls), the percent correctly classified by discriminant analysis was 79.41%. This change was not significant.

A second validation procedure was the examination of cases that were incorrectly classified by the discriminant analysis (i.e., the cases classified as false positive and false negative). These cases were traced in the original data and the circumstances surrounding these falls were analyzed.

Examination of the 17 controls who were classified in the fall group (i.e., as false positives) showed that six of these patients (35%)

were disoriented, all 17 (100%) had difficulty with balance, and 16 of the 17 patients had an abnormal gait (three patients were rated as "weak" and 13 as "impaired"). Only three of these patients used walking aids, and one ambulated by leaning on the furniture. Ten weeks later, the charts of these patients were obtained from the record department and examined for the possibility of falls that may have occurred after data collection had been completed. In that period, three of the 17 patients had fallen (one patient three times) for a total of five falls.

Twenty-two patients who had fallen were not classified in the fall group (i.e., were false negatives). Examination of these data showed that all patients were oriented, eight patients had a weak gait, and one an impaired gait. Only one patient used a walking aid. Examination of the falls experienced by these patients permitted classification into two types of falls: the unanticipated physiological fall ($n=8$) caused by "drop attacks," drug reactions, fainting, seizures, or patients with knees that "gave way," and the accidental fall ($n=14$), which included patients who slipped, tripped, or "rolled out of bed" (see Morse et al., 1987).

A third method of validation was the prospective testing of the *Scale* in three types of clinical settings: an acute care hospital (six units), long-term care (a psychogeriatric unit and a nursing home), and eight adult units in a rehabilitation hospital) (Morse, Black, Oberle, & Donahue, 1989). All patients ($n=2689$) were assessed daily for fall risk using the *MFS*. Differences in the distribution of scores were obtained by setting, 19.6% scoring high risk of falling in the acute care area, 45.1% in the long term care area, and 57.6% in the rehabilitation hospital. The *Scale* appeared sensitive to changes in the patients' conditions, with differences in the daily mean score between the long-stay and the short-stay patients and among surgical, medical, rehabilitation, and nursing home units.

In the study period, 147 falls were experienced by 107 patients. Of these falls 6.8% of the patients scored as low risk of falling, 16.3% as moderate risk, and 76.9% as high risk of falling. Of these 147 falls, 61.9% were physiologically anticipated falls (i.e., falls that occur when the patient is disoriented, has a weak or impaired gait, and uses a walking aid), 20 (13.6%) were unanticipated falls (i.e., falls that occur in patients who are usually oriented, who have drop attacks, or feel dizzy or faint), and 35 (24.5%) were scored as accidental falls (i.e., falls that are caused when the patient slips, trips, or rolls out of bed). Of the 113 falls where the patients were rated as high risk of falling, 82 (72.6%) were physiologically anticipated falls.

| B | # The *Morse Fall Scale:* Determining Level of Risk |

When using the *Morse Fall Scale* (MFS) *the level of risk* (or the cut-off score) that determines the percentage of patients who will receive intervention strategies must be adjusted to suit the patient population. As health care institutions are usually sorted into units and according to level of care and patient diagnoses, the risk of falling varies markedly from area to area. For instance, in an acute surgical ward, where the average length of stay is usually less than 120 days and the patients are ambulatory shortly following surgery, the number of falls reported is less than in a geriatric medical unit, and the mean fall score for the unit would be lower than the mean score for the geriatric unit.

This variation poses a problem when determining the high risk score for the institution. If the score is set low enough to detect all the possible falls in the surgical unit (e.g., 25), then almost all the patients in the medical unit will score above 25. As a result, the nurses would have to classify all the geriatric medical patients as at high risk of falling—in short, the *Scale* loses its "discriminating power." As some patients are more likely to fall than others, there will be too many false positives (see Morse, 1986).

Selecting a uniform higher value does not solve the problem, for then patients on the surgical ward who are likely to fall will be judged not at risk (i.e., the *Scale* will give too many false negatives). Thus, determining the score that will indicate high risk must be determined *by unit* in institutions where the patient population is diverse.

Administrators must recognize that setting the *Scale* too low, too conservatively, is costly—for fall prevention strategies will be implemented by too many false negatives—that is, for patients who are less likely to fall. Nurses will consider the *Scale* obscure and not bother to use it. Setting the level of risk at too high a level will result in patients being unprotected, falling, and injuring themselves—that is, there will be too many false negatives. At no time should the high risk score be more than 55; otherwise too many patients at risk of falling will be unprotected.

A second consideration is that the mathematical solution may not be the optimal clinical solution, for the mathematical model does not consider the ethical-moral consequences of an incorrect decision, of the risk of injury to unprotected patients. Again, using the data presented here, at no time should high risk be greater than 55.

CALCULATING RISK

Method One

The first principle is to recognize that the *Scale* does not predict all fallers with 100% accuracy. The *Scale* will only predict 82.9% of fallers, the physiological anticipated falls from a normal hospital population. When these data are placed on a graph and the level of high risk moved above 25, the percentage of false negatives (i.e., fallers who will be classified as nonfallers) increases (see Figure B.1). However, the percentage of nonfallers identified as at risk of falling will decrease. Conversely, if the level of risk score is moved toward zero, all the falls will be detected (i.e., the false negatives will not be a problem), but a high percentage of nonfallers will be classified as fall-prone (i.e., the percentage of false positives will increase).

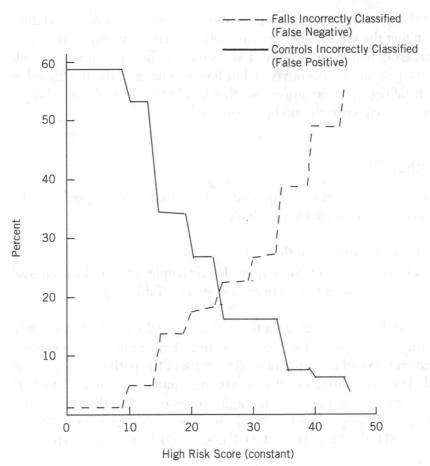

Figure B.1 Number of Falls and Controls Incorrectly Classified for Different Settings of the *Scale*

Note that the scores on Figure B.1 range to 50, while the *Scale* itself ranges up to 125. At no time should the high risk be set above 55, because the possibility of a false negative (i.e., considering a fall-prone patient at not at risk of falling—and therefore not providing fall intervention strategies) becomes too high. A survey conducted by Higley et al. of all patients in the VA system on the Eastern seaboard of the United States on 1 day revealed a greater percentage of patients at high risk of falling. Altering the cut-off score to a higher number does not change the percentage of patients who require surveillance. Rather changing the cut-off score places patients unnecessarily at risk. The increasing acuity of patients has increased the percentage of fall-prone patients in recent years, but has not changed the likelihood of their falling. It is recommended that in addition to high risk, the patient's actual score should be recorded.

Method Two

The method is a more subjective method that is often preferred by clinicians. The steps are as follows:

1 Score all patients in the unit.
2 List the scores by increment. For example, in a 34-bed surgical unit, the scores may appear as shown on Table B.1.

The staff may elect to set the high score at 25, in which case, 38% of the patients would be scored as not at risk, and fall prevention strategies would be implemented for 62% of the patients scored as at risk. However, the range of scores is large, and they may wish to "set" risk at two levels, medium and high. In this case, "medium risk" may be 25 to 45 (13 patients) and high risk, above 45 (8 patients). AT NO TIME SHOULD THE HIGH RISK SCORE BE SET HIGHER THAN 55.

Variation in the distribution of scores by acute care, long-term care or rehabilitation setting are presented in Appendix D, Table D.2, and may be used as a reference for determining the cut-off score. Note that in the total scores for this study, 52.5% of the scores were 25 or below, yet in the long-term care setting, only 20.1% of the scores were in this range.

VALUING THE COST OF AN INCORRECT DECISION

As stated, administrators must also consider the impact of the cost of a fall prevention program on hospital resources. Setting the "at-risk"

Table B.1

DISTRIBUTION OF FALL SCORES IN A SAMPLE UNIT

FALL SCORES	NUMBER OF PATIENTS	CUM %
0	6	18
10	2	24
15	3	32
20	2	38
25	2	44
30	3	53
35	5	68
40	1	71
45	2	76
50	2	82
55	1	85
60	1	88
65	0	88
70	1	91
75	1	94
80	0	94
85	1	97
90	0	97
95	1	100
100	0	
105	0	
110	0	
115	0	
120	0	

score too high will result in fallers being classified as nonfallers. If an injury occurs, it could legally jeopardize the institution. On the other hand, setting the risk score too low will result in too many patients at very low risk of falling being classified at high risk of falling, resulting in wasted staff time. It may even place the fall prevention program in jeopardy. Staff will rightly consider using the fall *Scale* "silly" if all patients are going to be rated at risk.

There is yet another consideration. The consequences of not identifying a faller as fall-prone, thereby risking injury and legal liability, may be considered 10 times (or 20 times—the number is determined by the institution) worse than identifying a nonfaller as a faller. The former has human costs and possible legal costs, while the latter may require more staff time. This is the relative risk, and it is used to weight the group at risk.

In the illustration below (Table B.2), different cost plans are shown. COST I: the hypothesized group—a fall correctly identified and a control correctly identified were weighted as 0, not identifying a fall was weighted as +10, and a control identified as a faller as +1. This resulted in an increase in the minimal level of setting the risk score.

These cost models may be further plotted for various scores, as shown in Figure B.2. Note there is a best minimum cost for each model. For cost 1, this is 25 to 39, so a high risk score of 35 should be used. For the second cost estimation, where the cost of not identifying a fall-prone patient (false negative) is estimated at 50 times that of identifying a nonfaller as a faller, the minimum high risk score is 25. But if the cost estimated is 200 times greater for a false negative, the minimum cost is zero, all patients must be considered at risk of falling.

In summary, to retain the discriminatory power of the *Scale*, the risk score should be adjusted according to the patient population and the cost that administrators place on not identifying a fall. Previous scales have not been developed to identify the fall prone patient in high risk areas, such as long-term care. In geriatric or rehabilitation areas, all patients have scored "at risk of falling," therefore the use-

Table B.2

HYPOTHESIZED COSTS TO THE INSTITUTION[1] BASED ON VARIOUS ESTIMATIONS OF RISK

| | Hypothesized Weight | | | | LEVEL OF *SCALE* |
COST PLAN	FALL GROUP CORRECTLY IDENTIFIED	FALL GROUP IDENTIFIED AS CONTROLS	CONTROLS CORRECTLY IDENTIFIED	CONTROLS IDENTIFIED AS FALLERS	SCORE FOR HIGH RISK AT MINIMUM COST
COST 1	0	+10	0	+1	35
COST 2	0	+50	0	+1	25
COST 3	0	+100	0	+1	0

[1]Estimated using a normalized population of 100 falls and 4,000 controls.

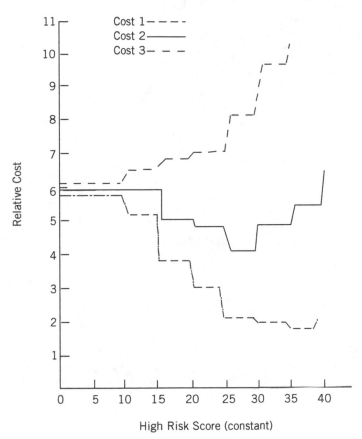

Figure B.2 Cost Estimates for Three Models with Different Settings of the High Risk Score (i.e., Constant)

fulness of identifying patients at risk is lost. In reality, all of these patients are at risk of falling. However, as clinicians are aware, some patients are more at risk than others; therefore, while precautions may be made with all patients, relative risk may also be measured and extra precautions targeted toward those patients most at risk.

REFERENCES

Morse, J. M. (1986). Computerized evaluation of a scale to identify the fall prone patient. *Canadian Journal of Public Health,* 77 (Supp. 1), 21–25.

A Comparison of Methods for Calculating Fall Rates

Fall rates have been difficult to compare because there is no established standard for reporting fall statistics. Without such a standard, hospitals have been forced to use a variety of different reporting conventions. This appendix discusses the various methods of reporting fall statistics and the strengths and limitations of each. Data used in this analysis were obtained from a prospective study that examined the identification of fall-prone patients in three settings—acute care, long-term care, and rehabilitation—at two institutions (Morse & Morse, 1989). The rates for the acute care institution were obtained from six patient care units (medical and surgical), where the patients were considered at a higher risk of falling than the total hospital population. These rates, therefore, are higher than normally reported. The long-term care sample consisted of one psychogeriatric unit and one 75-bed unit in a male nursing home. The rehabilitation sample was obtained from eight adult units in a rehabilitation hospital. Data for these three settings were collected over 6 months, from November 1985 to April 1986. Historical controls, obtained from hospital records for the same period in the previous year, are presented for comparative purposes. Table C.1 presents the data from this study.

Table C.1

DATA OBTAINED FROM A PROSPECTIVE STUDY EXAMINING THE IDENTIFICATION OF FALL-PRONE PATIENTS IN THREE SETTINGS

	Data Used in Analysis of Fall Rates			
	Area			
VARIABLES FOR STUDY PERIOD (1986) AND PREVIOUS YEAR (1985)*	ACUTE CARE *n*	LONG-TERM CARE *n*	REHABILITATION *n*	TOTAL *n*
Patient falls				
1985	55	35	52	142
1986	48	41	58	147
Patients who fell**				
1986	39	25	39	103
Patients who were injured				
1986	13	8	20	41
Patients at risk				
1986	1,939	124	626	2,689
Patient bed days				
1985	16,380	13,413	17,796	47,589
1986	16,563	13,542	19,841	49,946
Mean length of stay (days)				
1986	10	—	40	N/A

*For 6-month period, includes repeated falls by the same patient
**One fall recorded per patient

PATIENT FALL RATES

Health care institutions calculate the patient fall rate as:

$$\frac{\text{the number of patient falls}}{\text{number of patient bed days}} \times 1{,}000$$

Data are collected over a set period of time. Note that *all falls* are included in this formula, not all *patients who have fallen,* so that repeated falls are included in this formula. For these three settings during the study period of 1986, the fall rate can be calculated as 2.90 per 1,000 patient bed days for the acute care institution, 2.92 for the rehabilitation hospital, and 3.03 for the long-term care area. The fall rate for the three areas combined is 2.94 per 1,000 patient bed days.

THE NUMBER OF PATIENTS AT RISK

The second most commonly used statistic is the

$$\frac{\text{number of patient falls}}{\text{number of patients at risk}} \times 1,000$$

Because all institutionalized patients theoretically are at risk of falling, the number of patients at risk equals the number of patients admitted during the study regardless of their length of stay. "At risk" in this context does not refer to risk factors contributing to a fall. This method, as with the patient fall rate, includes the multiple, or repeated, falls, of any patient in the numerator. This may artificially inflate the statistics if there is a patient on the unit who falls frequently. The inclusion of multiple falls may give unstable or fluctuating rates over time. This is particularly important if falls are being monitored over a short period of time, such as when the administrator is working with monthly totals. Using the statistic from Table C.1 for 1986, we have the following:

$$\frac{147}{2689} \times 1,000 = 54.67 \text{ per } 1,000 \text{ patients at risk}$$

As mentioned, if a unit sometimes has a patient who is repeatedly falling and uses this statistic over a short period of time, such as the monthly monitoring of a unit, then this statistic may provide very unstable results. Differences between the *number of patients falls* and the *number of patients who fall* should be evident.

THE NUMBER OF PATIENTS WHO FELL

When the *number of patients who fell* is used as the numerator, rather than the *number of falls* per se, the fall rate is:

$$\frac{103}{2,689} \times 1,000 = 38.3 \text{ per } 1,000 \text{ patients}$$

THE NUMBER OF FALLS PER BED

This statistic is as follows:

$$\frac{\text{number of patient falls per time period}}{\text{number of beds}}$$

The potential problem with this method is that it gives no information about the length of time the patients are at risk and is based on the unrealistic assumption of 100% occupancy rate. Therefore, this statistic is dependent on the characteristics of the patient population; it is of limited use for comparison between units. For example, if the institution has long-stay patients, one would get results similar to the *number of patients at risk* if there was no patient turnover during the study period. On the other hand, if used for an acute care unit with short-stay patients, there would be a large discrepancy between these two results. Also note that *all falls* are included in this formula, not just the *number of patients who have fallen*.

THE PROBABILITY OF FALLING

This formula is useful, for it estimates the probability of any one patient falling on any 1 day:

$$\frac{\text{Fall rate}}{1,000}$$

Thus, based on the fall rate for the rehabilitation unit of 2.9 per 1,000 patient bed days, there is a 1:345 chance of a patient falling on any given day.

The reason why the formula yields only an estimate of probability has to do with more than just sampling variability. Because the falls counted in the fall rate include those from multiple fallers, patients who have been counted only once will be calculated to have a higher fall probability than should be the case.

If one wishes to calculate the probability of falling during an average hospital stay, it is not quite accurate to multiply the probability for a single day by the number of day's stay. If the duration were long enough, such a calculation would produce a "probability" greater than one, which is meaningless. The correct calculation is done by subtracting the probability from one to get the chances of *not* falling per day, then raising that value to the power given by the number of days, and finally subtracting the result from one again.

Thus, in the rehabilitation unit, with a fall probability of 0.0029 and a mean stay of 40 days, we would calculate:

$$[1-(1-.0029)^{40}] = [1-.9971^{40}] =[1-.8903] =0.11$$

which means there is approximately an 11% chance of falling during a stay in the rehabilitation unit.

REFERENCES

Morse, J. M., & Morse, R. M. (1988). Calculating fall rates: Methodologic concerns. *Quality Review Bulletin: Journal of Quality Assurance, 14*(12), 369–371.

D

Prospective Testing of the *Morse Fall Scale*

The purpose of this study was to clinically validate the *Morse Fall Scale* (*MFS*) in three types of patient care areas (acute medical and surgical units, long-term care areas, and a rehabilitation hospital). Patients' fall risk was rated daily and falls that occurred were analyzed by type of fall and risk score to determine the feasibility of using the *Scale* in practice.

METHOD

Setting

The study was conducted in two institutions. Six units were selected from the acute care division (general surgical [two units], ophthalmology [one unit] and three medical units), along with two units from the long-term care division (psychogeriatric and nursing home) in a 1,100-bed general hospital. Also eight adult units were selected from the 240-bed rehabilitation hospital (i.e., neuromuscular, orthopedic, diabetes, weight control, head injury [two units] and a CVA unit). The average length of stay in the acute care areas of the acute care hospital was 10 days, with a fall rate of 2.5 falls per 1,000 patient bed days calculated from the previous year. Patients were frequently transferred to the rehabilitation hospital from other hospitals in the region, and the average length of stay in that hospital was 40 days. The patient fall rate for the rehabilitation hospital for the previous year was 3.2 falls per 1,000 patient bed days.

Research Design

A pilot project to assess the feasibility of the project was initiated in November 1985. The pilot was conducted for 2 weeks to determine the most effective methods of data collection. Thereafter, one unit in each institution was introduced to the project every few weeks. For the first 1 or 2 weeks, staff were introduced to the project, instructed in the use of the *MFS* (from a video learning tape), and fall-prevention strategies were discussed. Nurses rated all patients' risk of falling daily, documented fall prevention strategies used and, if a fall occurred, noted the time of occurrence, type of fall, and any causative factors. Only falls that occurred on the patient's unit were included in the analysis (i.e., patient falls that occurred in another department, such as x-ray, or while the patient was out on a pass, were excluded).

RESULTS

Data collection extended from December 1, 1985, to April 30, 1986. A total of 252 weeks of data were collected from 16 patient care units. Of the 2,689 patients assessed during this period, 41.2% were over the age of 65 years; pediatric patients were excluded. Patients, by unit and gender are shown in Table D.1. A total of 49,946 patient bed days were recorded: 16,563 from the acute care areas, 13,542 from the long-term care areas, and 19, 841 from the rehabilitation hospital. As patients usually were not discharged from the hospital until they could cope without surveillance, the mean length of stay in each institution was used as an indication to compare the short- and the long-stay patients. The mean length of stay was 10 days in the acute care hospital

Table D.1

PATIENT GENDER BY UNIT						
	MALE		**FEMALE**		**TOTAL**	
UNIT	*n*	**%**	*n*	**%**	*n*	**CUM %**
Acute Care						
Ophthalmology	143	49.1	148	50.9	291	10.8
General Surgery I	115	49.8	116	50.2	231	8.6
General Surgery II	146	54.7	121	45.3	267	9.9
General Medicine I	260	54.5	217	45.5	477	17.7
General Medicine II	139	59.4	95	40.6	234	8.7
G.I. & Endocrinology	205	46.7	234	53.3	439	16.3
Long-Term						
Long-Term Care	13	28.3	33	71.7	46	1.7
Nursing Home	78	100.0	0	0.0	78	2.9
Rehabilitation						
Neuromuscular	19	44.2	24	55.8	43	1.6
Head Injury I	15	16.7	75	83.3	90	3.3
Orthopedics	84	94.4	5	5.6	89	3.3
Diabetes	39	60.0	26	40.0	65	2.4
Weight Control	28	31.5	61	68.5	89	3.3
Head Injury II	25	39.7	38	60.3	63	2.3
Stroke I	50	37.3	84	62.7	134	5.0
Stroke II	35	66.0	18	34.0	53	2.0
Total	1394	51.8	1295	48.2	2689	100.0

Those patients under 18 years of age were excluded from the research project because (1) regulation for the protection of Human Subjects requires parental consent for the inclusion of minors in research and (2) falls by young children include falls from climbing and tripping which are a part of normal activity and thus are considered a separate phenomenon.

and 40 days in the rehabilitation hospital. However, the mean length of stay could not be calculated for the long-term care area as the patients are rarely discharged.

Of 2,689 patients in both institutions, 1,265 (47.1%) scored as low risk of falling (i.e., ≤ 20), 734 (27.3%) scored as medium risk (i.e., 25–40), and 690 (25.5%) as high risk (i.e., ≥ 45). The distribution of total fall scores obtained by setting are shown in Table D.2. Distinct

Table D.2

FALL SCORES BY SETTING

FALL SCORE	Setting								
	Acute care		Long-term care		Rehabilitation		Total		
	n	%	*n*	%	*n*	%	*n*	%	CUM. %
0	522	26.9	3	2.4	27	4.3	552	20.5	20.5
10	37	1.9	0	0.0	14	2.2	51	1.9	22.4
15	241	12.4	22	17.7	57	9.1	320	11.9	34.3
20	332	17.1	0	0.0	10	1.6	342	12.7	47.0
25	63	3.2	4	3.2	81	12.9	148	5.5	52.5
30	99	5.1	11	8.9	22	3.5	132	4.9	57.4
35	197	10.2	16	12.9	49	7.8	262	9.7	67.1
40	66	3.4	12	9.7	114	18.2	192	7.1	74.2
45	75	3.9	0	0.0	6	1.0	81	3.0	77.2
50	75	3.9	17	13.7	91	14.5	183	6.8	84.0
55	41	2.1	1	0.8	15	2.4	57	2.1	86.1
60	45	2.3	7	5.6	26	4.2	78	2.9	89.0
65	20	1.0	9	7.3	39	6.2	68	2.5	91.5
70	35	1.8	0	0.0	2	0.3	37	1.4	92.9
75	25	1.3	13	10.5	52	8.3	90	3.4	96.3
80	7	0.4	1	0.8	6	1.0	14	0.5	96.5
85	20	1.0	0	0.0	0	0.0	20	0.7	97.5
90	6	0.3	7	5.6	13	2.1	26	1.0	98.5
95	13	0.7	0	0.0	1	0.2	14	0.5	99.0
100	6	0.3	0	0.0	0	0.0	6	0.2	99.2
105	3	0.2	1	0.8	1	0.2	5	0.2	99.4
110	5	0.3	0	0.0	0	0.0	5	0.2	99.6
115	0	0.0	0	0.0	0	0.0	0	0.0	99.6
120	0	0.0	0	0.0	0	0.0	0	0.0	99.6
125	1	0.1	0	0.0	0	0.0	1	0.0	99.6
Missing	5	0.3	0	0.0	0	0.0	5	0.2	99.8
Total	1939	100.1	124	99.9	626	100.0	2689	99.8	100.0

differences in the distribution of scores between groups were immediately apparent. The mean score in the acute care setting was 24.78 (*s.d.* 22.95), with 58.3% scoring as low risk, 21.8% as medium risk, and 19.6% as a high risk. In the long-term care setting, a mean score of 44.37 was obtained (*s.d.* 23.35); 20.1% of these patients received a low score, 34.7% a medium score, and 45.1% a high score. The scores for the rehabilitation area, with a mean of 41.9% (*s.d.* 21.11), showed that 15.6% rated low, 25.8% medium, and 57.6% as a high risk.

Analysis of each item in the *MFS* showed that 50.4% of the patients' scores varied during the hospital stay. The items that increase the mean scores were attributed to changes in ambulatory aids (30.1%) and deterioration in gait from normal to weak or weak to impaired (23.4%). A fall increased the patient scores in only 12% of the cases. On the other hand, a decrease in patient scores resulted from improvement in gait in 43.1% of the cases, the removal of an IV in 23.9%, and an improvement in mental status in 18.1%.

In the acute care setting, differences in fall scores according to patient condition were reflected when the scores of the short-stay (i.e., ≤10 days) and the long-stay (>10 days) patients were compared. When analyzed day by day, changes in the patients' scores reflected differences in the patients' condition (see Figure D.1). For example, many patients are admitted to the eye unit for minor surgery. The pattern of patient scores in this unit peak on the day following surgery (Day 2) for those admitted for minor surgery, and the scores decrease when these patients begin to ambulate as they approach discharge. On the other hand, the scores remain elevated for longer term patients. Unfortunately, the mean length of stay of 40 days did not provide an adequate sample to permit analysis between long- and short-stay patients in the rehabilitation hospital or for the long-term care setting. However, daily patient scores in the rehabilitation hospital did increase the second day after admission, perhaps because after assessment the patients were no longer on bed rest and were encouraged to ambulate. Nevertheless, in both the rehabilitation and the long-term care areas, scores were relatively flat compared with the variability evident in the acute care hospital.

Examination of the type of patient fall (i.e., physiological anticipated fall, physiological unanticipated fall, and accidental fall) by the patients' fall scores revealed that of 147 falls, 91 (i.e., 61.9%) were physiological anticipated falls, whereas only 20 (13.6%) were unanticipated falls and 36 (24.5%) were accidental. The largest percentage of fallers, regardless of type, were high scorers (76.9%); this difference was particularly apparent in the anticipated physiological fall category. The association between fall score category and type of fall

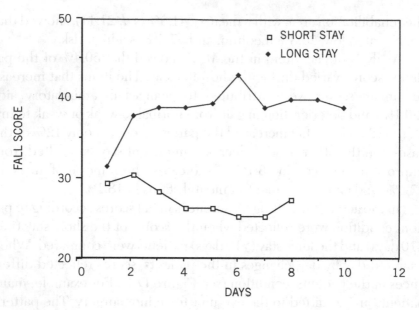

(i) Medical Units

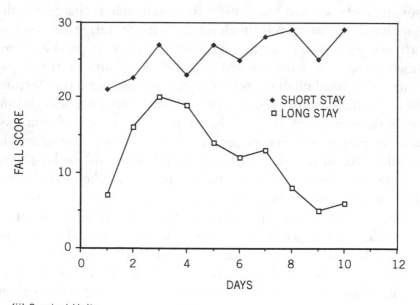

(ii) Surgical Units

Figure D.1 Daily Variation in Patient Fall Scores (i) Medical Units and (ii) Surgical Units

Table D.3

FALLS SCORE BY TYPE OF FALL AND SETTING

FALL SCORE	Anticipated $(n = 91)$[1]			Unanticipated $(n = 20)$[1]			Accidental $(n = 36)$[1]			Total	
	A/C[2]	LTC[3]	R[4]	A/C	LTC	R	A/C	LTC	R	*N*	%
Low	0	0	1	5	0	0	2	1	1	10	6.8
Moderate	4	2	2	1	1	3	2	5	4	24	16.3
High	26	25	31	3	1	6	5	6	10	113	76.9
Total	30	27	34	9	2	9	9	12	15	147[5]	100.0

[1] Number of falls
[2] Acute care
[3] Long-term care
[4] Rehabilitation
[5] Includes repeated falls (*n*=107 patients)

was statistically significant ($C^2 = 30.2$, *d.f.* = 4, p< .01) (see Table D.3). On the other hand, most of the falls with patient scores in the low or moderate categories were classified as "unanticipated" or "accidental" falls.

Of the patients who fell and were injured, the greatest proportion of injuries were incurred by those patients scored as likely to have "anticipated physiological falls" (i.e., 22 of 91 falls, or 24.2%). Of these, 8 of 22 falls resulted in serious injuries (see Table D.4). The only other serious injury in the study was an accidental fall, also experienced by a patient with a high fall score, who fractured both a hip and an elbow. Thirteen patients from the acute care area, 8 from the long-term care and 20 from the rehabilitation areas received injuries resulting from the fall.

Repeated Fallers

During the study period, 26 patients fell twice or more for a total of 66 falls (i.e., 26 first falls and 40 repeated falls), with one patient falling five times in the study period. The number of falls by patient care area

Table D.4

INJURIES BY SCORE AND TYPE OF FALL

FALL SCORE	ANTICIPATED (n = 91)[1]	UNANTICIPATED (n = 20)[1]	ACCIDENTAL (n = 36)[1]	TOTAL (n = 147)[1]
Low	0	2 minor	2 minor	4
Moderate	1 serious[2]	3 minor	3 minor	7
High	13 minor	5 minor	1 serious[4]	30
	8 serious[3]		3 minor	
Total	22	10	9	41

[1]Number of falls
[2]1 fracture ankle
[3]2 fractured ribs; 1 fractured hip; 1 fractured ankle; 1 fractured vertebrae (C2); 1 laceration; 1 sprain; 1 concussion
[4]1 fractured hip and elbow

Table D.5

NUMBERS OF PATIENTS WHO FELL REPEATEDLY, BY SETTING AND NUMBER OF FALLS

NUMBER OF FALLS	Setting		
	ACUTE CARE	LONG-TERM CARE	REHABILITATION
2	7	5	6
3	1	0	2
4	0	2	2
5	0	1	0
Total	17	23	26 = 66

are shown in Table D.5. The mean fall score for patients in this category was 80 (*s.d.* 17.6).

All of the scores of patients who fell repeatedly in the rehabilitation hospital are shown by fall in Table D.6. In this group, the scores of 6 of the 10 patients increased considerably over the course of hospitalization. Three of the patients in the acute care hospital also had

Table D.6

FALL SCORES FOR PATIENTS WHO FELL REPEATEDLY: REHABILITATION HOSPITAL

	Fall			
PATIENT	FIRST	SECOND	THIRD	FOURTH
1	50[a]	105[a]		
2	90[a]	90[a]		
3	65[ab]	90[ab]		
4	35[b]	75[b]		
5	75[b]	75[b]		
6	25[b]	40[b]		
7	75	75[ab]	75[ab]	
8	75[b]	75	75[b]	
9	60[b]	60[b]	90[b]	90
10	40[b]	65[b]	75[b]	90

[a] Same circumstances at time of fall (e.g., going to the bathroom)
[b] Same activity at time of fall (e.g., transferring or reaching for an object)

increased scores with subsequent falls, but the patients in the long-term areas, with higher mean scores, tended to have scores that were more stable.

At the conclusion of the project, the nursing staff was surveyed to ascertain the clinical feasibility of continuing the use of the *Scale*. Of the 175 nurses who responded, 82.9% rated the *Scale* as quick and easy to use, and 54% estimated that it took less than 3 minutes to rate a patient using the *Scale*. Sixty-three percent thought it should be a part of ongoing nursing assessment.

DISCUSSION

Longitudinal evaluation of the *MFS* shows that the *Scale* appears to be a valid predictor of patient falls. Of the total of 107 patients who fell during the study period, 113 of the falls were experienced by the 75 patients who scored in the "high-risk" category. The *Scale* was particularly successful in predicting anticipated physiological falls; 90.1%

of fallers in this category were identified by the *Scale* as being at high risk. Furthermore, the *Scale* is sensitive to changes in the patient condition, as evidenced by the variability in daily scores, particularly in the surgical areas of the acute care hospital. Items that contribute to the patients' fall scores vary by unit (i.e., by medical specialty), which suggests that the *Scale* is sensitive to levels of disability. There are distinct differences in the score profiles according to institution, with a greater proportion of patients receiving a high score in the long-term care institution and the rehabilitation hospital. Thus, the *Scale* is correctly identifying differences that are intuitively obvious; one would expect rehabilitation and long-term care patients to be at greater risk of falling.

It is important to note that although more than 57.6% of the rehabilitation hospital patients scored as having a high risk of falling, the fall rate (2.7 falls per 1,000 patient bed days) was lower than in the long-term care area and the acute care area (3.0 and 2.9 falls per 1,000 patient bed days respectively). All but one of the serious injuries occurring during the study period were in patients who were identified by the *Fall Scale* as being at high risk of falling. This suggests that patients in the high-risk category were more likely to be injured if they do fall and indicates that those caring for the patients with a high fall score should be increasingly aware of the necessity of fall prevention.

Examination of the scores of the patients that fell repeatedly showed that the scores were very high, and in nine cases, the scores increased substantially with each successive fall, indicating increasing frailty. This is consistent with other research (Gryfe, Aimes, & Ashley, 1977) which notes that falls tend to cluster prior to death.

There were two limitations to this study. First, the patient care areas were not selected randomly. They were chosen because they were considered "high-risk" areas, where patient falls were problematic. Thus, areas such as obstetrics were excluded, and the sample was not representative of a typical hospital population. Patients under the age of 18 years were also excluded, and no data are available on children or younger adolescents. It is recommended that the study be repeated, and *all* patients in several institutions be scored so that more representative norms of patient scores may be obtained.

The second limitation is a problem that is unavoidable when studying patient falls, and it is related to research design. It is not feasible to separate the rating of fall risk from the subsequent possibility of a fall without also trying simultaneously to prevent the fall. Thus, the researcher is in the paradoxical situation of both predicting the criterion variable and preventing its occurrence. There is, however, no moral solution to this problem, and it becomes a choice of conducting imperfect research or not conducting the research at all (Robb, Stegman, & Wolanin, 1986). Thus, the staff were given fall prevention strategies to prevent falls in patients rated at medium or high risk of falling despite the fact that successfully preventing a fall could interfere with the significance of the results.

A related problem with the researcher's or administrator's sudden interest in falls is the increased reporting of falls during a study period. As all patient falls that result in injury are reported, it is probable that injury rate is less variable to reporting error than fall rate. It is recommended that in future studies the injury rate during the research period be compared with previous years to identify changes in the standards of reporting.

Nevertheless, the major strengths of this project were that the study was conducted in the clinical areas during normal working days, and the ratings were done by clinicians who would normally be using the *Scale*. As other fall scales have been too complex to use without pencil and paper (Rainville, 1984) and required a physical examination (Tideikssar & Kay, 1986) or taking a clinical history (Patel, 1976) to assess the patient's fall risk, the ease of use and administrative feasibility of the *MFS* appears advantageous. However, although the *Scale* assists in the prediction of fall-prone patients, investigation of methods to prevent patient falls must continue.

REFERENCES

Gryfe, C., Aimes, A., & Ashley, M. (1977). A longitudinal study of falls in an elderly population: I. Incidence and morbidity. *Age and Ageing, 6,* 201–210.

Morse, J. M., Black, C., Oberle, K., & Donahue, P. (1989). A prospective study to identify the fall-prone patient. *Social Science in Medicine, 28*(1), 81–86.

Patel, K. P. (1976). Accidents in the home: Falls and faints in the elderly: Look to their clinical history for clues. *Modern Geriatrics, 6,* 28–34.

Rainville, N. (1984). Effect of an implemented fall prevention program. *Quality Review Bulletin, 9,* 287–291.

Robb, S. S., Stegman, C. E., & Wolanin, M. O. (1986). No research versus research with compromised results: A study of validation therapy. *Nursing Research, 35*(2), 113–118.

Tideikssar, R., & Kay, A. D. (1986). What causes falls? A logical diagnostic procedure. *Geriatrics, 41*(12), 32–50.

Problems in Evaluating Fall Risk Scales

The intent of research-related fall risk prediction scales is to develop an instrument that will quickly triage those who are at risk of falling, thereby enabling preventive and protective strategies to be immediately put in place to prevent patient injury and to monitor fall risk throughout their hospital stay. Before continuing with the discussion, however, it is important to differentiate fall risk prediction scales (instruments intended to identify the fall prone and to *predict the risk of falling*), from instruments that are used for patient *assessment,* that is, to assess the individual's *condition* (usually physiological-based factors) that may cause a patient fall, such as gait assessment. *Assessment instruments* are time consuming to use, but provide information about the nature of physiologically based deficits so they can be rectified before a fall occurs (i.e., fall preventive measures, such as exercise or balance training programs, to improve gait). By extension they may also assist in identifying the need for fall protective strategies (such as a hip protector to prevent a fractured hip should a fall occur). For example, a fall risk prediction scale might rate gait as normal, weak, or impaired, according to gross indicators based on mobility, while assessment instruments would require actual measurement of strength, balance, and so forth. Note that risk prediction scales provide patient scores that indicate risk of falling, but do not tell us why or what to do to prevent the fall, just as a thermometer will tell us if the patient has a fever, but not what is causing the fever or how it should be treated.

Altman (1997) noted the tension between the purposes of these two types of instruments in trying to "reconcile pragmatism with methodological purity" (p. 1309): clinicians expect risk prediction scales to provide prescriptive information about fall prevention strategies, so they are tempted to add variables that provide diagnostic validity. But adding variables not only invalidates the scale's performance, but also moves the purpose away from fall *risk prediction* toward *fall assessment*. Recently, for instance, McFarlane-Klob, (2004) published a *"Modified Morse Scale"* (without consulting the developer) and added medication variables. If this researcher had understood how the *MFS* was developed and how it worked, she would have known that medications were evaluated during the scale construction. Furthermore, making the scale longer defeats the purpose of efficient rating and does not increase the validity of the scale.

METHODS OF SCALE DEVELOPMENT

Fall prediction scales "work" because researchers have developed both the items and the item scores (the weights for those items) in an exploratory process by comparing a large number of variables that may possibly contribute to a fall in subjects who *have fallen*, compared to those who have *not* fallen. This comparison of groups enables the identification of items that are statically significant. Computer modeling should be used in an exploratory manner, combining variables to form indices, hence enabling the identification of the minimal number of variables to eventually constitute the scale items, without reducing the ability of the scale to differentiate the fall group from the control. Next, statistical weights of the significant items may be converted to produce item scores, and the scale is subsequently modeled in the data set to assess validity, performance, and cut-off scores to determine levels of risk. Of course, these statistical weights as they are first calculated are not likely to be whole numbers and would not be practical for use in the clinical setting. In the *Morse Fall Scale* (MFS), these numbers were rounded to the next whole number divisible by five, and then the discriminant function of the scale was recalculated to ensure the scale still worked.

This method of scale construction has been used with only two scales—the *MFS* (Morse, Morse, & Tylko, 1989) and the recent modification of the STRATIFY tool (Oliver, Britton, Seed et al., 1997) in Hamilton, Ontario (Papaiannou, Parkinson, Cook et.al., 2004). The Hendrich II (Hendrich, Bender, & Nyhuis, 2003) approximates this approach, but it is not clear how the scores were calculated from data presented, why all significant items were not included in the final scale, and if the final scale was subsequently clinically tested.

However, most of the fall risk prediction scales available do not follow this design. Some have been developed using a control group to identify statistically significant items, but with the item scores arbitrarily assigned (e.g. *Downton Index* [Vassallo, Vignaraja, Sharma et al., 2004]; STRATIFY scale [Oliver, Britton, Seed et al, 1997]). In addition, some scales used retrospective chart reviews as data rather than as patient assessment (e.g., the *Scott and White Falls Risk Screener* [Yauk, Hopkins, Phillips et al., 2004]), hence limiting variables that could be identified as significant. Furthermore, some researchers have selected scale items using techniques of *face validity*, which is considered atheoretical, imprecise, and the weakest of all validities (Newfields, 2002). Using their own clinical judgment, these researchers have selected items by surveying other scales for the items most frequently used or have selected those that they consider, from their own clinical experience, may cause a fall. Some of these instruments are simply checklists (e.g., Haines, Bennell, Osborn, & Hill, 2004; no author, 2000); others have arbitrarily assigned scores to the items—scores also based on the researcher's own judgment and convenience. These values are often 1s, 2s, and 3s selected for the clinicians' ease for totaling the scores, and the resulting scores are used to determine classes of high or low risk of falling (e.g., Browne, Covington, & Davila, 2003). (Note that when easily added numbers were assigned to the *MFS*, the discriminant function went down to .5 [or to the same ratio that one would obtain by flipping a coin]. It is **both** the combined function of item selection *and* the weight of the score assigned to the item that makes the *MFS* valid.)

Another criterion of validity of risk prediction scales is that they must work clinically. Scales must be sensitive to patients' conditions by providing a range of scores (the *MFS* is scored 0 to 120) and also be sensitive to the individual patient's change in condition. Finally, they must have been tested independently by another institution. This criterion was met by McCollam (1995) for the *MFS*.

Often these poorly constructed scales are used internally by hospitals. Some have been published (e.g., Brown, Covington, & Davila, 2003; Dempsey, 2004; Hathaway, Walsh, Lacy, & Saenger, 2000; Udèn, Ehnfors & Sjostrom, 1999), others disseminated via the Internet (Farmer, 2000). These scales are usually "tested" in the clinical area by noting the fall score of the patients who actually fall: If the score of the patient who falls is in the estimated "high-risk" range, then the scale is considered the scale to "work" and is declared valid. However, except at a very gross or obvious level, if tested correctly with a control group, these scales probably will not differentiate the fall-prone patients from those who are not fall-prone. Of greatest concern, these instruments do not have the refinement to be able to accurately predict the fall-prone patient, and worse, have not been finely tuned to minimize the false negatives—that is, patients who are actually at risk of falling are not identified. Hence, these scales may have little validity or psychometric standardization (Perell, 2002).

The cost of using poorly constructed scales clinically is in the number of false negatives (or rating a patient *not at risk* when the patient actually *is fall-prone*) is very high, thus risking not identifying patients in need of fall protective and preventive strategies and placing the patient at risk of injury should a fall occur. *This is the most serious consequence of "homemade" instruments.* The quality of homemade scales is poor and the safety of patients may be jeopardized. Given the availability of scales with diagnostic accuracy, there is no need for facilities to develop their own scales (Perell, Nelson, Goldman et al., 2001).

Why do clinical nurse researchers go to all of the trouble and expense of developing a homemade scale, when scales with reliability and validity data are available? Some nurse researchers have reviewed the *MFS* and determined that it was not generalizable for their context. I am puzzled by such comments as "it was developed on Canadians" or "not suitable for our Australian context" (McFarlane-Kolb, 2004), because the MFS does not contain contextual variables.

Another problem is that in the development of these scales, specialized patient populations are used. For instance, the STRATIFY scale was developed using elderly patients from three hospitals (Oliver, Britton, Seed et al., 1997). In the development of the MFS, patients were also recruited from three hospitals: acute care, rehabilitation, and nursing home hospitals. Although we deliberately tried to make a scale that was valid for all patients, we did not include outpatients, day surgery, psychiatric, or home care patients. There is no theoretical rationale however, why the scale will not perform for these groups, and it would be faster to develop normative scores for those populations, than to develop another scale.

MODELS USED TO EVALUATE FALL RISK SCALES

Unfortunately, researchers have caused harm by inaccurately or improperly evaluating fall risk scales. As a consequence of these errors, excellent research is devalued and even debunked, and research gains are lost. Worse, some of these reviews have been published, so that rather than using completed research, the research effort, of varying quality, has continued in search of a reliable means to predict fall-proneness. The problems of the evaluation research include (1) inappropriate design used for clinical testing, and (2) errors in evaluation.

INAPPROPRIATE DESIGN USED FOR CLINICAL TESTING

Once a scale is developed, it is tested for clinical feasibility. Two problems of invalidity have emerged, affecting both homemade scales and those developed more rigorously. These are the Hawthorne effect and the disregarding of interventions that form intervening variables between obtaining the patient's fall score and the opportunity for a fall to occur.

The Hawthorne Effect

Clearly, simply implementing a fall intervention program may alter the fall rate: (1) staff previously casual about reporting falls may now conscientiously report every fall, causing the falls rate to increase (see, e.g., O'Connell & Myers, 2001); and (2) staff are more aware of falls risk and may adopt falls prevention strategies, causing the falls rate to decrease. Therefore fall rates may be unreliable, and the fall *injury* rate is a more valid statistic for evaluating the efficacy of the fall intervention program. Nurses always file a fall incident report when a patient is injured, but because injury is a relatively rare event, this may also be unstable for statistical reasons.

Problems of Design of Clinical Trials

Researchers often use the number of falls and the fall scores of the patients who fall to assess the efficacy of the risk prediction scale. But the number of falls *evaluates the fall intervention program, not* the efficacy of the scale. Once a patient is rated at risk of falling, staff members are obligated to implement fall prevention strategies that actually stop the patient from falling. Therefore, these intervention variables interfere with the measurement of the dependent variable and invalidate the trial to the extent that it is unreasonable to use these numbers to ascertain the sensitivity and specificity of a fall risk scale. Implementing such research design is akin to developing a Suicide Prediction Scale and administering it to all pedestrians who walk on to a bridge. Because the bridge is a favorite place from which to leap, barriers have been erected, video surveillance alert guards, and the police prevent anyone for climbing on to the bridge railing to leap; hence, no one is able to commit suicide regardless of intent. Does this mean there is anything wrong with the Suicide Predictor Scale? No— the intervening variables interfere with the relationship. Understandably, using a similar research design for determining the validity of a fall risk scale will not provide meaningful information about the validity of the scale. Yet researchers have done this and published their results in refereed journals—and even wondered why their results obtained from using the *MFS* are at variance with those originally reported (see, for instance, O'Connell & Myers, 2001, 2002).

ERRORS IN EVALUATION

Faulty methods of evaluation have also been used. These include the reliance on face validity, failure to use the original publications when assessing performance, and trialing scales against each other and with nurses clinical judgment.

Reliance on Face Validity

These review articles present tables listing all of the scales and comparing the items in each scale (Evans, Hodgkinson, Lambert, & Wood, 1998, 2001; The Joanna Briggs Centre; Morse, 1993) to determine whether they "fit" some preconceived domain of factors that cause patient falls. Note that the value assigned to each item in the respective scales is omitted from these tables, so that the comparisons are meaningless.

Failure to Use the Original Source When Assessing Performance

A review is valid only if it is complete. Yet in the review of fall risk scales reported by The Joanna Briggs Center (Australia) (Evans, Hodgkinson, Lambert et al., 1998), this was not the case. Instead of using the publication reporting the *MFS* development (i.e., Morse, Morse, & Tylko, 1988) they used a publication describing the characteristics of types of falls (Morse, Tylko, & Dixon, 1987). This is a surprising error for the original source is cited in many earlier publications, and the research program is even summarized in a book (Morse, 1997). Given their omission of key publications, one must challenge Evans, Hodgkinson, Lambert et. al.'s (1998) strong conclusion that "Falls risk assessment tools are very inaccurate. . . . no evidence to suggest that the generic risk tools . . . offer any additional benefits over tools that are used within a single institution and have been developed based on that population's characteristics . . . no particular risk assessment tool can be assessed" (p. 30).

Trialing of Scales Against Each Other and With Nurses' Clinical Judgment

Some researchers have trialed risk assessment scales against nurses' clinical judgment and, when finding neither excellent, have recommended the use of a combined approach (both the scale and clinical judgment) (Moore, Martin, & Stonehouse, 1996). However, these trials are inadequately designed. Researchers did not control for nurses' prior knowledge about falls or knowledge of fall assessment. Of greater concern, in the study by Eagle, Salama, Whitman et al. (1999), which tested three methods of assessment—nurses clinical judgment, the Functional Reach Test to measure balance (Duncan, Weiner, Chandler et al. (1990), and the MFS—the researchers used the MFS incorrectly, scoring the patients using retrospective chart review rather than assessing them (Eagle et. al., 1999). The MFS cannot be validly completed by using chart data—patients *must* be examined— but these evaluators did not do this. Further, while the raters and the nurses were blind to the patients' MFS scores, it was not known if raters (who were using their clinical judgment) had used the MFS and/or other methods to rate patient risk of falling previously. In other words, there was no control over the nurses' knowledge about fall risk assessment. Was their clinical judgment blind to research knowledge? This threat to validity would be very difficult to control.

INVALID DESIGN OF CLINICAL TESTING

The most problematic design of fall intervention program research is the simultaneous testing of the fall risk prediction scale and the fall interventions. O'Connell & Myers' (2001) study used this design, but it was further confounded by a second fall intervention study conducted simultaneously, but unknowingly, by the occupational therapy staff. Despite these problems (which included the intervention program interfering with their dependent variable, the fall rate), they were still critical of the predictive validity of the MFS (O'Connell & Myers, 2002). Their false positive rate (i.e., 79% of patients rated at risk of falling and who did not fall), perhaps meant that their interventions were working, not that the scale was problematic with limited generalizability, as they concluded (p. 135).

How did we therefore obtain sensitivity and specificity statistics for the MFS that apparently cannot be replicated? First, we studied patients who fell *at the time of the fall (confirmed fallers)* and controls—those who had *not* fallen, and this provided sensitivity of 78% and specificity of 83% (Morse, Morse, & Tylko, 1989). These results were satisfactory, but were still not without problems, for there were a number of errors—false positives (patients who had not fallen who were considered by the computer to be at risk) and false negatives (patients who had fallen and were rated as not at risk). We investigated these errors by examining the charts of these patients 10 weeks after the initial analysis. We found that the false positive group had a high rate of falls (five of the 17 patients had fallen; one patient fell three times) and concluded the computer was correct—these patients were at risk but had not had the opportunity to fall before the time of the original data collection, and they increase the sensitivity of the scale to 91%. The falls that were experienced by patients who rated at risk of falling by the MFS, we labeled *physiological anticipated falls.* Next, by examining the circumstances of falls that occurred in patients in the false negative group, we identified two additional types of falls: the accidental fall (true accidents, slips, and trips in those who are rated at not risk of falling) and the unanticipated physiological falls (falls due to a seizure or fainting in patients who also scored not at risk) (Morse, Tylko, & Dixon, 1987). Recalculating the ability of the scale to discriminate after making these corrections, the sensitivity and specificity of the scale increases to 84% sensitivity. But the importance of recognizing the three types of falls is that the scale will never identify 100% of falls in a hospital, and staff members should always try to determine what type of fall occurred, record statistics accordingly, and be aware that the preventive and protective strategies for each type of fall differs (Morse, 1997). The site of accidental falls must be investigated to prevent recurrence, and strategies implemented to protect those with unanticipated falls from injury should a second fall occur.

CLINICAL ERRORS WHEN USING THE SCALE

Essential to the clinical performance of a scale is its correct use in patient assessment. This assessment is reasonably quick for the *MFS* (it takes 1 to 3 minutes), but users need to have received instruction.

Not Using the *MFS* According to Directions

As noted above, the lack of correct assessment and inaccurate scores results in errors. Despite the availability of instructional tools for the *MFS*, some clinicians do not realize that scoring the patient requires patient examination. As with all forms of assessment, if the scale is not used correctly, regardless of its reliability and validity, it will not perform as expected clinically. Patient safety will be jeopardized.

Failure to Acknowledge the Sensitivity of the Scale

The second problem occurs when the staff record the patient's score as *high risk* or *low risk* and do not record the total score (Perell, Nelson, Goldman et al., 2001). This is akin to recording a patient's temperature as high or low without recording the actual figure, so that staff does not know if the temperature is increasing or decreasing or the severity of the fever. Similarly if the actual fall score is not recorded, then staff does not know how high the fall risk is and whether it changes throughout the 24 hours. As the goal of care is to reduce the score, if the actual score is not recorded, then it will not be possible to gauge improvement (and decrease of fall risk) or an increasing score (and therefore increased risk of falling).

"All Patients Scored at High Risk"

A frequent complaint is that all of the patients scored high risk of falling—that is, the scale does not discriminate adequately. It is possible that all of the patients are, for instance, at high risk. Raising the level of risk will not change this fact and will place those who are at risk in the "not at risk" category (i.e., a false negative). But if each patient's actual score is recorded, then the staff will recognize that there are discernable degrees of high risk.

Infrequent Scoring

The final problem is not scoring the patient frequently enough. An emerging standard is that patients should be scored upon admission, and thereafter if a patient's condition changes. This is not frequent enough for patients in acute care, who should be scored at least once per shift. In long-term care, where patient fall risk is more stable, the patients should be scored frequently over several 24-hour periods until their pattern is recognized, and then less frequent scoring—as infrequently as once a week—if the resident's condition remains stable.

DISCUSSION: SO WHAT? WHAT IS AT RISK?

Given the poor quality of this clinical evaluation research and unrealistic expectations of the scale's performance, it is not surprising that the quest for a perfect—or at least improved—scale has continued since the development of the *MFS*. Patient falls is probably one of the most researched clinical problems in nursing. The responsibility for patient falls has been placed squarely on the shoulders of nursing. We feel guilty if a patient falls, blaming ourselves for not remaining vigilant and perhaps even for neglecting basic care. ("I should have asked this patient if she needed toileting.") Because of this firm link to basic nursing skills, many nurses have attempted to examine the problem of falls in various ways. Researchers are motivated by clinical *problems*—they hope interesting problems—those that will improve nursing care and change patient outcomes. Thus patient falls has been researched and researched by nurses, and this research continues to the present time.

However, the research is extraordinary. Each project is conducted in relative isolation from other projects, so that the research is not cumulative overall. Project after project is conducted with the aim of developing yet another fall risk prediction instrument. The failure to utilize the work of others has "leveled the playing field" and often results in mighty steps backward. The problem is compounded by invalid methods of evaluating and testing the available instruments, as well as a lack of rigorous, funded inquiry by experienced researchers.

Review articles, including the Cochrane reviews, do link fall research, but these are not without error and omissions—which are then perpetuated by means of meta reviews (see, e,g,, Burrows, 1999).

Astonishingly, this research is by and large being conducted using "opinion," albeit under the guise of clinical judgment. The Cochrane criteria are correct: Opinion (be it "clinical judgment," "intuition," or "expert committee decisions") results in poor research involving measurement and in a low level of evidence. In the case of nursing fall research, this overreliance on soft data results in the paradox of applying "qualitative" data to a quantitative problem. It is the poorest of qualitative work, inappropriately applied, with the results masquerading as a quantitative tool that jeopardizes patient safety. Patients risk injury—and even death.

Safety research is important, but it must be safe. It must be given adequate funding, conducted by researchers with appropriate qualifications, implemented wisely, and evaluated appropriately. Fall risk prediction is not easy to research; the outcome variable is intercepted; fall risk changes rapidly, and—particularly in the acute care setting—is unstable, so that frequent assessments are essential. Fall intervention programs are not a low-cost add-on in the clinical area; they are expensive in time and dollars, but are essential to safe care. Fall risk assessment is a task that can be achieved only through the education of nurses, some time commitment in their workload, some attention by the quality assurance department to the recording of scores and fall statistics, and some investment on the part of administration for program costs. Fall intervention programs require all of these commitments, plus funding of a position for a clinical specialist to organize the program, funding for fall prevention and protection devices, funding to ensure that the building and equipment are as safe as possible, and vigilance and responsiveness to the program as a whole. Without the complete package, fall injuries in hospitals will not be reduced.

REFERENCES

Altman, D. G. (1997). Study to predict which elderly patients will fall shows difficulties in deriving and validating a model. *British Medical Journal, 315,* 1309.

Browne, J. A., Covington, B. G., & Davila, Y. (2004). Using information technology to assist in redesign of a fall prevention program. *Journal of Nursing Care Quality, 19*(3), 218–225.

Burrows, E. (1999). *What strategies exist for the effectiveness of fall preventions strategies of older patients in institutional settings?* Clayton, Victoria, Australia: Centre for Clinical Effectiveness, Monash University. Retrieved October 10, 2005, from *http://www.med.monash.edu.au/healthservices/cce/evidence/pdf/b/234.PDF*

Camicioli, R., & Licis, L. (2004). Motor impairment predicts falls in specialized Alzheimer care units. *Alzheimer Disease and Associated Disorders, 18*(4), 214–218.

Charting tips: Documenting a patient's fall risk. (2000). *Nursing, 30*(11), 14.

Dempsey, J. (2004). Falls prevention revisited: A call for a new approach. *Journal of Clinical Nursing, 13,* 479–485.

Duncan, P. W., Weiner, D. K., Chandler, J., & Studenski, S. (1990). Functional reach: A new clinical measure of balance. *Journal of Gerontology, 45,* M192–M197.

Dyer, A. E., Taylor, G. J., Reed, M., Dyer, C. A., Robertson, D. R., & Harrington, R. (2004). Falls prevention in residential care homes: A randomized controlled trial. *Age and Ageing, 33,* 596–602.

Eagle, D. J., Salama, S., Whitman, D., Evans, L. A., Ho, E., & Olde, J. (1999). Comparison of three instruments in predicting accidental falls in selected inpatients in a general teaching hospital. *Journal of Gerontological Nursing, 25*(7), 40–45.

Evans, D., Hodgkinson, B., Lambert, L., Wood, J., & Kowanko, I. (1998). *Falls in acute hospitals: A systematic review.* Adelaide, Australia: Joanna Briggs Institute for Evidence Based Nursing and Midwifery.

Evans, D., Hodgkinson, B., Lambert, L., Wood, J., & Kowanko, I. (2001). Falls risk factors in hospital settings: A systematic review. *International Journal of Nursing practice, 7,* 38–45.

Farmer, B. C. (2000, May). Fall risk assessment. *Try This: Best Practices in Nursing Care to Older Adults, Hartford Institute for Geriatric Nursing, 8.* Retrieved October 16, 2005, from *http://www.hartfordign.org/publications/trythis/issue08.pdf*

Haines, T. P., Bennell, K. L., Osborne, R. H., & Hill, K. D. (2004). Effectiveness of targeted falls prevention programme in subacute hospital setting: Randomised control trial. *British Medical Journal, 328*(7441), 676.

Hathaway, J., Walsh, J., Lacey, C., & Saenger, H. (2000). Insights obtained form an evaluation of a falls prevention program set in a rural hospital. *Australian Journal of Rural Health, 9,* 172–177.

Healey, F., Monro, A., Cockram, A., Adams, V., & Heseltine, D. (2004). Using targeted risk factor reduction to prevent falls in older in-patients: A randomized controlled trial. *Age and Ageing, 33,* 390–395.

Hendrich, A. L., Bender, P. S., & Nyhuis, A. (2003). Validation of the Hendrich II Fall Risk Scale: A large concurrent case/control study of hospitalized patients. *Applied Nursing Research, 16*(1), 9–21.

Joanna Briggs Institute. (1998). Falls in hospitals. *Best Practice: Evidence based Practice information sheet for Health Professionals, 2*(2), 1–6.

McCollam, M. E. (1995). Evaluation and implementation of a research-based falls assessment innovation. *Nursing Clinics of North America, 30*(3), 507–514.

McFarlane-Klob, H. (2004). Falls risk assessment: Multi-targeted interventions and the impact on hospital falls. *International Journal of Nursing Practice, 10,* 199–206.

Moore, T., Martin, J., & Stonehouse, J. (1996). Predicting falls: Risk assessment tool versus clinical judgment. *Perspectives, 20*(1), 8–11.

Morse, J. M. (1993). Nursing research on patient falls in health care institutions. *Annual Review of Nursing Research, 11,* 299–326.

Morse, J. M. (1997). *Preventing patient falls.* Thousand Oaks, CA: Sage.

Morse, J. M. (2002). Enhancing the safety of hospitalization by reducing patient falls. *American Journal of Infection Control, 30*(6), 376–380.

Morse, J. M., Morse, R. M., & Tylko, S. J. (1989). Development of a scale to identify the fall-prone patient. *Canadian Journal on Ageing, 8*(4), 366–377.

Morse, J. M., Tylko, S. J., & Dixon, H. A. (1987). Characteristics of the fall-prone patient. *Gerontologist, 27*(4), 516–522.

Newfields, T. (2002). Challenging the notion of face validity. *JALT Testing and Evaluation, 6*(3), 19–20.

O'Connell, B., & Myers, H. (2001). A failed fall prevention study in an acute care setting: Lessons from the swamp. *Interntional Joural of Nursing practice, 7,* 126–130.

O'Connell, B., & Myers, H. (2002). The sensitivity and specificity of the Morse Fall Scale in acute care settings. *Journal of Clinical Nursing, 11,* 134–136.

Oliver, D., Britton, M., Seed. P., Martin, F. C., & Hopper, A. H. (1997). Development and evaluation of evidence-based risk assessment tool (STRATIFY) to predict which elderly patients will fall: Case control and cohort studies. *British Medical Journal, 31,* 1049–1053.

Oliver, D., Daly, F., Martin, F., & McMurdo, M. E. T. (2004). Risk factors and risk assessment tools for falls in hospital in-patients: A systematic review. *Age and Ageing, 33,* 122–130.

Papaioannou, A., Parkinson, W., Cook, R., Ferko, N., Coker E., & Adachi, J. D. (2004). Prediction of falls using a risk assessment tool in acute care. *BMC Medicine.* Retrieved November 1, 2005, from *http://www.biomedcentral.com?17417015/2/1*

Perell, K. L. (2002). Assessing the risk of falls: Guidelines for clinical practice settings. *Generations, 3,* 56–59.

Perell, K. L., Nelson, A., Goldman, R. L., Luther, S. L., Prieto-Lewis, N., & Rubenstein, L. Z. (2001). Fall risk assessment measures: An analytic review. *Journal of Gerontology. Series A: Biological Sciences and Medical Sciences, 56A*(12), M761–766.

Undén, G., Ehnfors, M., & Sjostrom, K. (1999). Use of an initial risk assessment and recording as the main nursing intervention in identifying risk of falls. *Journal of Advanced Nursing, 29*(91), 145–152.

Vassallo, M., Vignaraja, R., Sharma, J. C., Hallam, H., Binns, K., Briggs, R., Ross, I., & Allen, S. (2004). The effect of changing practice on fall prevention in a rehabilitative hospital: The Hospital Injury Prevention Study. *Journal of the American Geriatrics Society, 52*(3), 335–339.

Yauk, S., Hopkins, B. A., Phillips, C. D., & Bennion, J. (2005). Predicting in-hospital falls: Development of the Scott and While Falls Risk Screener. *Journal of Nursing Care Quality, 20*(2), 128–133.

F

Translations of the *Morse Fall Scale*

DANISH VERSION

Morse Fall Scale		Score

1. Anamnese:
   Er indlagt p.g.a. fald eller faldet
   inden for de seneste 3 måneder.
	Nej = 0
	Ja = 25	

2. Har patienten mere end een diagnose	Nej = 0 Ja = 15	
3. Har patienten brug for hjælp til mobilisering	Fast sengeleje, kørestol, personalestøtte = 0 Stok, gangstativ = 15 Støtter sig til møbler = 30	
4. Har patienten IV-adgang(e)	Nej = 0 Ja = 20	
5. Hvordan er patientens gang / forflytningsevne	Normal, fast sengeleje, immobil = 0 Let kompromitteret = 10 Kompromitteret = 20	
6. Hvordan er patientens mentale status	Orienteret i egne data, tid og sted = 0 Glemmer egne begrænsninger = 15	
	Total score	

Translation by Lotte Evron

Risiko niveau	MFS Score	Handlinger
Ingen risiko	0-24	Ingen
Lav risiko	25-50	Gå til: Procedurer ved Standard fald-forebyggelse
Høj risiko	> 50	Gå til: Procedurer ved Høj risiko fald forebyggelse

SPANISH VERSION

Escala de Morse Nivel de Riesgo de Caídas		
Aspecto a valorar	Ingrese "S" ó "N"	Valor
1. Historia de caídas; 0 a 3 meses	N	25
2. Diagnóstica Secundario:	N	15
3. Ayuda Ambulatoria		
a. Ninguna, Reposo Absoluto, Silla de ruedas,Asistencia de Enfermería	N	0
b. Muletas, bastón, caminadora.	N	15
c. Equipo especial de movilización	N	30
4. Sello de heparina, venoclisis	N	20
5. Traslado; seleccione uno de las siguientes opciones		
a.Normal, Reposo Absoluto, Inmovilizado	N	0
b.Ambulatorio.	N	10
c. Inquieto	S	20
6. Estatus Mental; seleccione una de la siguientes opciones		
a. Bien orientado	S	0
b. Desorientado	S	15
TOTAL		125
Nivel de Riesgo		0

Rango		Nivel de Riesgo
0	24	0
25	44	1
45	125	2

I thank César A. Cisneros Puebla, UAM Iztapalapa.

GERMAN VERSION

Morse Sturzskala

Bestandteil   *Punkte*
Eintrag

1. **Sturzgeschichte**   Nein   0   _____
                                                     Ja   25   _____

2. **Zweitdiagnose**   Nein   0   _____
                                                     Ja   15   _____

3. **Gehbehel**

   Kein/Bettlägerigkeit/Unterstützung durch Pfleger(in)   0
   _____

   Unteram-Stützkrücken/ Gehstock/Gehwagen, Rollator   15   _____
                   Möbel   30   _____

4. **Intravenöse Therapie / Saline-Schloss**   Nein   0   _____
                                                     Ja   20   _____

5. **Gang(art)**
        Normal/Bettlägrikeit/Rollstuhl   0
   _____

                Schwach   10   _____
                Beeinträchtigt   20   _____

6. **Geistiger Zustand**
        Richtige Einschätzung der eigenen Fähigkeiten   0   _____
        Überschätzt sich / vergisst Selbsteinschränkungen   15   _____

FRENCH VERSION

ÉCHELLE DE CHUTES MORSE – FORMULAIRE DE COLLECTE DE DONNÉES

Catégorie de l'échelle de chutes Morse	Circle/*Encercler* Yes/*Oui* No/*Non*	Score	Patient Score *Score du patient/de la patiente*
1. Patient has a history of falling Le patient/la patiente a des antécédents de chutes	No/*Non* Yes/*Oui*	0 25	
	No/*Non* Yes/*Oui*	0 15	
2. Patient has a secondary diagnosis *Le patient/ la patiente a un diagnostic secondaire*			
3. Patient uses ambulatory aid (*Le patient/la patiente utilise une aide à la marche*) none/bedrest/nurse assistant(*aucune/repos au lit/aide infirmière*) crutches/cane/walker (*béquilles/canne/marchette*) holds on to furniture (*se tient aux meubles*)	 Yes/*Oui* Yes/*Oui* Yes/*Oui*	 0 15 30	
4. Patient uses ambulatory aid (*Le patient/la patiente utilise une aide à la marche*) none/bedrest/nurse assistant(*aucune/repos au lit/aide infirmière*) crutches/cane/walker (*béquilles/canne/marchette*) holds on to furniture (*se tient aux meubles*)	No/*Non* Yes/*Oui*	0 20	
5. Patient's Gait/Transferring (*Démarche/Transfert du patient/de la patiente*) Normal/bedrest/immobile ((*normal/repos au lit/immobile*) Weak (*Faible*) Impaired (*restreint*)	 Yes/*Oui* Yes/*Oui* Yes/*Oui*	 0 10 20	
6. Patient's Mental Status (*État mental du patient/de la patiente*) Oriented toward own ability(*Connaît ses propres capacités*) Overestimates/forgets limitations (*Surestime/oublie ses limites*)	 Yes/*Oui* Yes/*Oui*	 0 15	

Risk Level *Niveau de risque*	Morse Fall Score *Score de l'échelle de chutes Morse*	Action *Mesures*
No Risk/*Aucun risque*	0-24	Universal Fall Prevention Interventions *Interventions universelles de prévention des chutes*
Low Risk/*Faible risque*	25 – 45	Fall Prevention Interventions *Interventions de prévention des chutes*
High Risk/*Risque élevé*	≥ 46	High Risk Fall Prevention Interventions *Interventions de prévention des chutes – situations à risque élevé*

Date: _____   Time/Heure:_____   Recorder's Signature/
Signature de la personne qui a rempli ce formulaire

Acknowledgement: Hôpital regional de Sudbury Regional Hospital

JAPANESE VERSION

日本語版 Morse Fall Scale

ID_____ 名前_____ 年齢_____ 性別（男・女） 日時_____

主病名_____合併症_____   評価者サイン_____

		ポイント	得点
1. 転倒歴	なし	0	_____
	あり	25	_____
2. 合併症	なし	0	_____
	あり	25	_____
3. 歩行補助具			
なし/ベッド上安静/看護師の補助		0	_____
松葉杖/杖/歩行器		15	_____
家具などの伝い歩き		30	_____
4. 静脈内注入療法/ヘパリンロック	なし	0	_____
	あり	20	_____
5. 歩行			
正常/ベッド上安静/車椅子		0	_____
不安定		10	_____
障害されている		20	_____
6. 精神状態			
自身の能力を判断できる		0	_____
過大評価/制限を忘れる		15	_____
		合計	_____

Morse JM, et al.: Can J Aging 1989; 8(4): 366-77より

リスク水準	合計点数
転倒リスクなし	0-24点
低い転倒リスク	25-44
高い転倒リスク	≥45

具体的対策

KOREAN VERSION

몰스 낙상 척도 (Morse Fall Scale)

구분	척도		대상자 점수
1. 낙상의 경험	없음	0	
	있음	25	
2. 2차적인 진단	없음	0	
	있음	15	
3. 보행 보조	보조기 사용하지 않음/와상/케어자가 도와줌	0	
	목발/지팡이/보행기	15	
	가구를 잡고 보행함	30	
4. 정맥 수액요법/헤파린 락 (Heparin Lock)	없음	0	
	있음	20	
5. 걸음걸이	정상/와상/부동	0	
	허약함	10	
	장애가 있음	20	
6. 정신상태	자신의 기능수준에 대해 잘 알고 있음	0	
	자신의 기능수준을 과대평가하거나, 한계를 잊어버림	15	
총점			

◇ 결과해석
  총점 0-24 낙상의 위험 없음.
     25-50 낙상의 위험 낮음.
     ≥51 낙상의 위험 높음.
  단 시설의 종류에 따라 절단점을 다르게 적용할 수 있음.

Source: Morse, J. M. (1997). Preventing patient falls. p41. Thousand Oaks, CA: Sage Publication, Inc. 원저자의 허락을 받고 김현숙이 번역함.
I thank Hee Yeon, Shin, Samsung Medical Center (SMC), Seoul, Korea.

MANDARIN VERSION

摩尔斯摔跌测试表

项目			得分
1. 摔跌史	无	0	
		25	———
2. 第二诊断	无	0	
	有	15	———
3. 行走辅助			
无/卧床休息/护士辅助		0	
拐杖/手杖/助行器		15	
扶靠家具行走		30	———
4. 静脉治疗/	无	0	
肝素锁	有	20	———
5. 步态			
正常/卧床休息/轮椅		0	
无力		10	
残疾		20	———
6. 精神状态			
量力而行		0	
高估/忽略能力限度		15	———
		总分	———

若得分超过 45 分则属高风险

I thank Betty Wills, RN, PhD.

FILIPINO VERSION

Morse Sukatan sa Pagkakahulog

Bagay-bagay sa Talaan			Puntos
1. Kasaysayan ng Pagkakahulog	wala	0	
	meron	25	____
2. Pangalawang Pagsusuri	hindi	0	
	oo	15	____
3. Tulong sa Paglalakad			
hindi makalagad/nakahiga/sa tulong ng tagapag-alaga		0	
saklay/tungkod/panglakad		15	
sangkapang panglakad		30	____
4. Bagbigay ng likido sa pamamagitan ng ugat/	hindi	0	
madaliang pagbigay ng IV	oo	20	____
5. Lakad			
karahiwan/nakahiga/sangkap panglakad		0	
mahina		10	
hindi karaniwan/maykapansanan		20	____
6. Kalagayan ng pag-iisip			
maymalay sa sariling kakayahan		0	
labis ang kalkula ng sariling kakayahan/		15	____
makalimutin sa sariling hangganan			
		Kabuuan	____

Mapanganib kung ang puntos ay ≥ 45
I thank Alberta Pasco, RN, PhD.

PERSIAN VERSION

<u>مقیاس اندازه گیری افتادن مورس</u>

	0	•	•
ندارد دارد	0 25		• • −1
ندارد دارد	0 15		• •−2
ندارد دارد	0 15 30		• • •• • -3 • / • / • • •• / / • •
ندارد دارد	0 20		• • - 4 دسترسی بورید
ندارد دارد	0 10 20		: -5 • •/ • / • ضعیف مشکل حرکتی
ندارد دارد	0 15		• •−6 / • • • • • • / • • •

I thank Shahnaz Moezzi, RN, PhD, University of Utah.

Index